# YOUR UCAS PERSONAL STATEMENT

# WHAT TO WRITE IF YOU WANT TO GET IN

**for Medicine, Dentistry, Veterinary Medicine, and Nursing**

**by**

**Gwyn Day**

**and**

**Chloë Daniel**

Published by gwynday.com, UK



ISBN: 978-0-9926649-9-2

# CONTENTS

# INTRODUCTION

## MY BACKGROUND

I am an educational coach specialising in beating admissions procedures. With 20 years of experience, I know what university admissions tutors are looking for. My expertise is in helping you give them what they want to win your place at your chosen university.

This is why the top fee-paying schools in the country (where parents pay annual fees of over £35,000) bring me in to talk to their students; it is why I am on the Supervisory Board of Oxbridge Applications and deliver training sessions to thousands of students every year; and it is why I am flown to India, Dubai, and Hong Kong to prepare individual private clients for their university and job applications.

The people I help fall into three main groups:

**Group 1:** Students with excellent grade profiles who want to get in for Medicine, Dentistry, Veterinary Medicine, or into Oxford, Cambridge, or US Ivy League colleges.

**Group 2:** Students who want to get into the best university possible given their grade profile.

**Group 3:** Undergraduates who want careers in Investment Banking, Management Consultancy, or Law (focusing on getting

Vacation Scheme placements and Training Contracts). For more details, see "The Programme" on my website www.gwynday.com and the book "Gwyn and The City - Commercial Awareness for Future Bankers, Lawyers, and Management Consultants" (available later this year).

If you are reading this book, the chances are you fall into **Group 1** (or **Group 2**). Welcome! Now let's move on to getting you into a great university.

Getting an offer from good universities depends on four (often five) factors:

1. Your GCSE grade profile (too late to worry about that)
2. Your AS results and predicted grades (that's your job)
3. Your Teacher's Reference (see Chapter 11)
4. Your Personal Statement - read on ...
5. Admissions tests (BMAT or UKCAT), interviews, and submitted work (see Chapter 14)

Here is some great news. If you follow all the guidance in this book, you will get an offer from one of your chosen universities (providing your AS grades match the university's requirements).

This book will help you write your own exceptional Personal Statement. Some students are looking for more one-on-one support. If you want me to advise, correct, edit, and proofread your Personal Statement unlimited times until you are happy with it, contact me via www.gwynday.com to arrange a chat.

## YOUR PERSONAL STATEMENT

Let's start with the basics. Your Personal Statement is part of your UCAS application and is submitted online along with your personal details, grade profile, and university choices.

For your Personal Statement, UCAS gives you 4,000 characters (including spaces). This roughly equates to one side of A4 paper. That is one side of paper to give the admissions tutors at your chosen universities enough evidence to show that you are smart, genuinely interested in your subject, understand the demands and benefits of the course, will contribute to the university, and, crucially, that you can write coherent, accurate, structured English.

A daunting prospect? This is much more straightforward than it sounds. The secret to success is knowing how to give the admissions tutors what they want - that means knowing how to match their idea of a great candidate.

My expert advice tells you how to do just that. With suggested reading, example paragraphs, practice exercises, and the lowdown on the main errors students make, the logical and detailed steps in this book will guide you through writing an exceptional Personal Statement that puts you ahead of the competition.

Follow all of the advice and you will get in. Do not cut corners.

## PLAGIARISM ALERTS

Throughout the book you will see the following warning written above sections that you are most likely to want to copy directly into your Personal Statement.

****PLAGIARISM ALERT****

Universities have plagiarism software to compare Personal Statements submitted this year with a huge database of those from previous years. This book, and others similar, will be scanned and added to their database. <u>If you copy, you will be caught</u>.

Help is at hand. Chapter 9 takes you through the different phrases, tweaks to word order, and bigger structural changes you can use to make your Personal Statement truly <u>yours</u>. This means that you get to use all the ideas in this book and still finish with a unique and effective Personal Statement.

## FAQs

### Question 1: When should I start writing my Personal Statement?

The best time to <u>finalise</u> your Personal Statement is immediately after your AS (or equivalent) results come in. By waiting until you get your AS (or equivalent) results, you will know which universities and courses will be relevant for you. It is all about being realistic. If your results are lower than expected, it will not make sense to apply to universities or courses with a high grade threshold. If your grades are better than expected, you may want to change your target universities and your course choice.

The period earlier in the summer, between finishing your AS exams and getting your results, is still crucially important. This is the perfect time to get your Personal Statement research done and start writing initial drafts.

The application deadline for Oxbridge, Medicine, Dentistry, and Veterinary Medicine is 15th October. There is only very limited term time left once you return from the summer holidays to get this done, so finalising your statement before you get back to school is essential to making it strong enough to stand out from the competition.

The Personal Statement Timeline in Chapter 1 shows you exactly what to do and when.

*(NOTE: If you decide to work with me on your Personal Statement one-on-one, we can start the process as soon as your exams are over. You get unlimited rewrites and checks, and, by starting early, I can guide you through the initial research.)*

## Question 2: How many drafts will it take to get my Personal Statement right?

If you want to produce a truly outstanding Personal Statement, in my experience you will be close to a final version within seven to ten drafts. Once you think you are close to a final version, you will realise one of two things. Either (1) you are well over the 4,000 character count and do not know what to take out because "it's all important", or (2) you have written more than half of your statement on extracurricular activities instead of detailing why you are the right candidate for your chosen course. Chapter 11 helps you fix these sorts of mistakes and turn your draft into its final, successful version.

## Question 3: How much time will it take me to write it?

Much longer than you think. Writing time will add up to somewhere between fourteen and seventeen hours. Before that, you will need time for research, extra reading, and online lectures, which, if done properly, could take you three to four days. A strong range of work experience is essential for Medicine, Dentistry, Veterinary Medicine, and Nursing applicants. Reading additional material related to the work experience you have already done, identifying what gaps you have, and then completing more placements to fill these takes more time still. The good news is that using this book will significantly reduce the amount of time required and give you a much better finished product.

## Question 4: Where do I start?

"I don't know how to start" is the most common concern I hear when working with students in schools, so you are not alone. Chapters 4, 5, 9, and 10 give specific ideas and phrase suggestions to get you started.

## Question 5: How do I know when my Personal Statement is finished?

As with any carefully crafted piece of writing, your Personal Statement is never finished. You can keep on replacing a word here or there, tweaking the word order, or finding another lecture or book that fits in with your interests. You must go for "optimum" rather than perfect.

Follow the advice in this book and your Personal Statement will be excellent. Then move on: concentrate on getting the grades at A2, and excelling at admissions tests and interviews.

## Question 6: I cannot fit in everything I want to say. How do I choose?

The art of writing an excellent Personal Statement is in choosing what is most directly relevant to demonstrate (not describe) your interest in your subject. Chapters 4, 5, 6, 7, and 8 take you through how to decide what is relevant and what is not.

Once you have established what you want to say, you then need to trim the word count. The exercises in Chapter 11 show you how to reduce the length of your statement without losing valuable content.

Remember a Personal Statement showing subject-specific reading, work experience, and other relevant, subject-specific activities, with only two lines on your "other hobbies", is fine; writing half (or more) of your Personal Statement on playing football and your band's latest gig is not.

**Question 7: I do not have any evidence to show why I am interested in the course. What should I do?**

You are set for a busy summer, but if you are applying for a subject which genuinely interests you the process of accumulating this evidence (though time-consuming) will be fun. To set about this as efficiently as possible, it is essential you read Chapters 4, 5, and 6 thoroughly. They detail easy ways to expand your reading and activities, and then how to work this evidence of your interest and motivation into your Personal Statement.

Being selective is key - otherwise you will be overwhelmed by new information. From my lists of suggestions (in Chapters 4, 5, and 6) pick only:

- two books (Chapter 4);
- two work experience placements (Chapter 5)
- three lectures from either TED or iTunes U (Chapter 5);

- one piece of archived material from the listed societies (e.g. Royal Society or Intelligence Squared) (Chapter 5).

Rather than overfilling your head with more information, take time to analyse and compare your selection cleverly. Do this, and you will be fine.

*(NOTE: If this is your situation, I strongly advise using my One-on-One Personal Statement Coaching. See www.gwynday.com for details.)*

**Question 8: I do not know why I want to study my chosen course - I just do. What do I write then?**

If you feel like this, you need to follow this book to the word. The examples given will provide you with many possible approaches and routes to take. Choose the approach which attracts you the most and you feel most comfortable with. Springboard off the examples given - especially in Chapters 4 and 5. By the end, you will definitely have some great reasons for your choice.

**Question 9: I want my Personal Statement to be unique. I'm worried it will be too formulaic if I use this book.**

There are only so many things that can be said in a Personal Statement (give me £1 for every time I read about Duke of Edinburgh's Awards or Grade 8 violin). A strong Personal

Statement is more about the “how” than the “what”. For good candidates, the “what” (e.g. books, activities, hobbies) is likely to be fairly constant. Most people do A-levels (or an equivalent), read around their subject, and have a few hobbies.

What differs is “how” you go about your Personal Statement. Have you given evidence rather than describing what you do? Have you been specific? Have you used a varied and intelligent writing style, and taken the time to ensure your Personal Statement is free of errors? These are the things that make a Personal Statement stand out.

The exercises in Chapters 9, 11, and 12 will help you turn your strong “core” Personal Statement into a captivating and unique one.

### Question 10: My teachers and others are giving different advice to you. Who is right?

Many great teachers, heads of sixth, and careers advisors know this process inside out. Look at the success rate certain schools have in getting their students into the top universities. Others do not, and that goes for parents too. They want to "help" but can sometimes end up causing confusion and weakening your application.

When you go to open days at your target universities or if admissions tutors visit your school, listen closely to what they say. Read all the free Personal Statement advice you can find online.

Then compare it to what I say and decide for yourself. Ultimately, it is your Personal Statement.

**Question 11: You mentioned that if my AS results are lower than expected I should avoid applying to certain universities or courses because their grade thresholds are too high. I am confident that I can improve at A2. Can I write my Personal Statement on that basis?**

There are two reasons why it is rare (though not impossible) for students to significantly improve on their AS results at A2: (1) A2 exams are much tougher than AS; and (2) the weighting of the marks allocated in AS/A2 makes it much easier to do well at AS.

For the vast majority of students I see, it is much more realistic to apply on the basis of AS results. If you do end up markedly improving at A2, you can always take a gap year and apply again the following year.

**Question 12: I would like to work with you directly. What do I do?**

Contact me via my website (www.gwynday.com), and I will be in touch to discuss rates and timeframes.

## Chapter 1

# PERSONAL STATEMENT TIMELINES

You are probably reading this book because you have just finished your AS exams and your teachers want you to start working on UCAS and your university application. The exact date you start this process will vary from school to school. To make it clear, I have set out a sequential timeline without fixed dates. This serves as a set of steps to follow from the moment you start.

Very few students will plan so far ahead that they are reading this earlier in Year 12, though as a prospective student for Medicine, Dentistry, or Veterinary Medicine with the early application deadline (15th October) and emphasis on multiple work experience placements, you certainly should be. The application deadline for Nursing is later (15th January); still, getting started early will ultimately result in a fuller and richer Personal Statement. If you want to be well organised, see the "Ideal Timeline" at the end of this chapter.

## SEQUENTIAL TIMELINE

### Step 1

Read this book all the way through and make no notes.

### Step 2

Read the book again.

**Step 3**
According to the different examples given in the chapters (e.g. books, lectures, extracurricular activities), make a list of everything you have done or been involved in so far which could be relevant for your statement.

**Step 4**
Identify the gaps. By that I mean work out what additional material you need to fully prove your suitability for your chosen course (e.g. one or two articles in subject-related magazines; a few TED talks or archived university public lectures; relevant work experience for the summer holidays).

**Step 5**
Complete or set up the extra work you identified in Step 4.

**Step 6**
Research your chosen courses and universities. Make notes about particular modules, course structure, opportunities (e.g. dissertation; time abroad; career opportunities), and the specific qualities they are looking for in candidates.

**Step 7**
Using the relevant chapters of this book to guide you, draft each paragraph of your Personal Statement in turn. It is fine for what you write to be rough at this stage; you will go on to revise each section many times. Your main focus here is getting down your information.

**Step 8**
Re-read the chapters relevant to each paragraph and use the information to improve the phrasing and particular words in your statement.

**Step 9**
Check your statement for "banned language", bad style, and overused clichés, as highlighted in Chapter 3, and replace with better expressions.

**Step 10**
Use Chapter 9 to edit, restructure, and refine your Personal Statement until you are confident that it feels truly yours.

**Step 11**
Check the length of your statement. Use Chapter 11 to make it more concise and Chapter 12 to weed out any final errors. Then complete this process again.

**Step 12**
Ask someone else to check the content and look for potential errors you have missed. Bear in mind, however, that you are going to receive advice from many sources (this book, teachers, your parents / guardians, university tutors coming into school, even online forums). Ultimately, you decide. It is your Personal Statement, nobody else's. Choose from all the advice and use what is right for you.

## IDEAL TIMELINE

If you have got yourself organised early in Year 12, or even in the summer between GCSEs and AS, you have lots of time to ensure you have all the evidence you need to write a truly outstanding Personal Statement. The following calendar timeline will guide you through the process.

### 1. Year 12: September / October

Start building evidence of your interest and motivation by:
(a) researching universities and courses;
(b) joining relevant clubs and societies at, or outside of, school;
(c) reading books and making notes;
(d) attending free public lectures and watching lectures online;
(e) setting up relevant work experience placements.

### 2. Year 12: March

Use this book to write the first draft of your Personal Statement. During this process, identify what gaps of knowledge or work experience you still need to fill.

### 3. Year 12: April / May

Revise: doing your absolute best in your AS exams is the most important thing right now.

### 4. Year 12: June, post-AS exams

Write draft 2 of your Personal Statement.

**5. Year 12: June / July**

Attend open days at the universities you are considering.

**6. Year 12: July / August**

Refine the material already in your statement and move towards a final draft.

(a) Work in relevant summer activity (e.g. summer schools, latest books, current affairs, recent work experience placements).

(b) Prepare for admissions tests and potential interviews.

(c) Check character count.

(d) Use the "Style Guide" in Chapter 3 to make sure your statement reads as fluently as possible.

(e) Check the proportion of subject-specific material is enough.

**7. Year 13: September 30th**

Final internal deadline, either for school or for you.

**8. Year 13: October 15th**

Oxbridge, Medicine, Dentistry, and Veterinary Medicine deadline.

**9. Year 13: December 1st**

Absolute last advised deadline for any Nursing applications.

**10. Year 13: January 15th**

Actual UCAS submission deadline.

## Chapter 2

# GETTING STARTED: PERSONAL STATEMENT OVERVIEW

Before you start writing your Personal Statement, or even doing the background research, it helps to have a sense of the basic structure you will use. Knowing what information you are ultimately aiming to include, and in what order, gives you an idea of where each paragraph is going and the purpose of your research.

### BASIC STRUCTURE

Your Personal Statement will consist of five paragraphs. At this early drafting stage, the five paragraph structure ensures that you include everything necessary to produce a robust final Personal Statement. Tweaks and styling can come later.

When you finally submit your statement via UCAS, it will flow as one single block of text. Doing otherwise is impossible because of the 4,000 characters limit. Despite this, you will still think of your statement in terms of clear paragraphs, each addressing a specific point.

Chapters 4, 5, 6, 7, and 8 in this book each tackle a separate paragraph, taking you through how to pull together and present the relevant material. Chapter 9 shows you how to give your Personal Statement the emphasis and narrative most important to you.

**Paragraph 1: Why this course**

Admissions tutors want you to prove that you are motivated to study your chosen course and that you have reflected on and understand why you want to study it. The five "big reasons" you can give are in Chapter 4. Whichever reason you decide on, ultimately important is showing that you have given solid thought to your decision.

**Paragraph 2: Examples of subject-specific further reading (i.e. not part of your obligatory A-level work)**

Having evidence of your interest in your subject beyond your A-level work is absolutely essential. This is how you can make your Personal Statement shine out among the many mediocre ones. You go to university to <u>read</u> a subject, so no surprise that you get bonus points for talking intelligently about the reading you have done off your own back at Sixth Form.

If you have not yet done any wider reading, Chapter 5 gives you plenty of ideas on where to start, including specific examples of books to mention in your statement and quotes you can use. Just referencing <u>two or three books</u> related to your areas of interest will put you <u>far</u> ahead of most candidates.

### Paragraph 3: Other <u>subject-specific</u> extracurricular activities

Without relevant and varied work experience, you stand little chance of getting in for Medicine, Dentistry, Veterinary Medicine, or Nursing. Showing you understand the daily challenges of the profession you are choosing is essential. Chapter 6 gives you a host of ideas for work experience is a must, and the many additional activities related to your subject which will help your statement stand out.

Showing how these experiences have deepened or sharpened your understanding of your subject - what admissions tutors expect - requires a great deal of thought. The examples in Chapter 6 show you how to do this effectively. Note that because work experience is so significant for your course, it is likely you will refer to placements in paragraph 2, in relation to your further reading or in their own right, and then refer to others in paragraph 3. As you will see from the example statements in Chapter 10, these two paragraphs will be relatively fluid in your final version.

### Paragraph 4: <u>Non subject-specific</u> extracurricular activities

Given the work experience requirement for your course, much of your statement will be taken up with subject-specific activities, leaving little space for other hobbies. That said, if you have taken something outside of school to a high level and, in doing so, have developed skills relevant to your chosen course, this are worth mentioning. There are multiple options to include here. Sports at international / national / county / school level; music; drama; having a part-time job; hobbies; Duke of Edinburgh's Award; School Council; Head Boy; Head Girl; Prefect; raising money for charity, the list goes on. Chapter 7 gives you ideas on what to include and how to present these succinctly to prove that you have what it takes, whilst leaving enough space for your other, more directly relevant activities.

**Paragraph 5: Wrap up**

In the fifth and final paragraph of your Personal Statement you will talk about what you want to gain from your degree and where you want it to take you (e.g. career / postgraduate study). Adding a personal comment that comes "from the heart" is a nice touch; so do mention, for example, that you are the first person in your family to go to university, that your family recently moved to the UK, or that English is your second language.

*NOTE 1: The first three paragraphs should make up approximately 85% of your Personal Statement (that equates to just over 3,500 characters including spaces).*

*NOTE 2: Teachers often instruct students to include details of what they have learned in their A-levels. Personally, I think (and the success of my clients has proven) that concentrating on evidence (of research, interest, ability, competence) rather than giving a descriptive statement regarding A-level content is much more effective in impressing admissions tutors. The examples below show you why.*

*Example -- okay but not ideal:*

“My four subjects at AS level have been very useful: Biology for an introduction to anatomy, Chemistry for practical laboratory skills, Maths for logic and problem-solving, and Geography for an understanding of cultural and social differences which influence attitudes to healthcare.”

*Example -- much better:*

“This degree course, according to your prospectus, values both practical research skills as well as a deep understanding of biomedical sciences. The former is shown by my EPQ on “The Health Impact of Sugary Drinks”, which combined controlled trials, statistical analysis, and wider independent reading. My gold medals in Chemistry and Biology Olympiads evidence the latter.”

## Chapter 3

# STYLE GUIDE

Expressing yourself intelligently is one of the best ways to make your Personal Statement stand out. To achieve this, thinking carefully about the style of writing you will use, before you start, is crucial.

The vast majority of the statements I see, including from top Oxbridge candidates, employ the same set of tedious stock phrases and fall into some very predictable language traps. Avoid these in yours and you will be far ahead of the competition.

Below I have highlighted the worst offenders. From now on consider these "banned style" and "banned words" to strictly avoid in your Personal Statement. Using the suggested alternatives will make a much better first impression.

## BANNED STYLE

### 1: Starting with a quote

Starting your Personal Statement with a quote is unimaginative and fails to show the admissions tutors anything other than your ability to use Google. Your Personal Statement is about why <u>you</u> want to do the course, not about some business guru, philosopher, or novelist.

Quotes can be appropriate elsewhere in your statement - see the examples in Chapter 5 (which guides you through writing paragraph 2). For this all important first line, however, a sentence about you and your motivation is much more effective.

A few of the worst offenders ...

| | |
|---|---|
| **Medicine** | "Wherever the art of medicine is loved, there is also a love of humanity." (Hippocrates) |
| **Medicine** | "Medicine is a science of uncertainty and an art of probability." William Osler |
| **Dentistry** | "For there was never yet philosopher that could endure the toothache patiently" William Shakespeare in "Much Ado About Nothing" |
| **Dentistry** | "Every tooth in a man's head is more valuable than a diamond." Miguel de Cervantes in "Don Quixote" |
| **Nursing** | "The very first requirement in a hospital is that it should do the sick no harm." Florence Nightingale |
| **Veterinary Medicine** | "I hope to make people realise how totally helpless animals are, how dependent on us, trusting as a child must that we will be kind and take care of their needs." James Herriot |

### 2: Describing

The purpose of your Personal Statement is to convince admissions tutors of your interest in and aptitude for your chosen subject. Using what you know and have done to show your suitability is far more interesting to them than a long-winded regurgitation of the university prospectus, your A-level syllabus, or a random list of your achievements. Clear points plus evidence are key.

*Example -- not so good:*

"Nursing is about caring and an interest in medical science." (So what. The tutor knows all of this and it says nothing about you.)

*Example -- better:*

"The combined experience of Biology A-level and volunteering at at a local nursing home has reinforced my commitment to Nursing as my future career."

**3: Poetry**

At best, overly flowery language is a waste of precious space, especially if combined with describing (see above). At worst, it makes you sound pretentious.

*Examples -- not so good:*

"To practise medicine in the NHS is to soothe the fevers and tend the wounds of a nation."

"I am a passionate science student and am fond of exploring the majestic landscapes of the small intestine."

*Examples -- better:*

“An important part of my motivation for studying Medicine at university is to work within the NHS and use this experience to ultimately help shape public health policy in Britain.”

“Exploring the functions of the small intestine by reading [XYZ] in my own time has made me realise how fundamental the digestive system is to good health and the research potential there is in this area.”

## 4: Egoism

Convince tutors that you are someone they want to teach, not someone so overconfident that you might not be willing to learn. Tell it like it is and always emphasise the relevance of your achievements for your course.

*Example -- not so good:*

"My great success at the Physics Olympiad, winning a gold medal for the second year running, shows that I am right for this course."

*Example -- better:*

“Working hard and independently preparing for the Physics Olympiad was rewarding, especially when I won the gold medal (for the second year,) and gives a good foundation for university-level work."

### 5: Extreme sentencing

Clear writing comes from clear thinking. If you find yourself writing in long, complicated sentences, it is likely that you have not yet worked out exactly what it is you want to say. Take a moment to think before you start writing to be sure of the purpose of each sentence. Then make your writing as concise as you can and punctuate properly (see Chapters 11 and 12).

*Example -- not so good:*

"Reading about what the author perceives to be the health impact of high-fructose corn syrup in "Why We Get Fat" by Gary Taubes, which he thinks makes the body go into insulin production overdrive and is ultimately one of the biggest causes of obesity epidemic started in the second half of the twentieth century, made me think about parallel developments in dental health across the developed world from North America to Europe and what impact this might have on the developing world as they shift towards a more Western-style diet."

*Example -- better:*

"After reading "Why We Get Fat" by Gary Taubes, I have been analysing the impact of the increased consumption of high-fructose corn syrup (HFCS) on dental health. The ideas Taubes puts forward about HFCS's role in the obesity epidemic of the late twentieth and early twenty-first century made me think that there must have been parallel devastating effects on people's teeth, and that this should be factored into public health plans in the developing world as people adopt more Western-style diets."

### 6: Phrase / word repetition

So many of the statements I review use the same phrase over and over again. It makes the ideas sound dull, even if they are not. Common offenders are:

- "led me to"
- "allowed me to"
- "gave me an understanding of"
- "gave me an insight into"

Carefully review what you have written, and where you see repetition use synonyms (see the examples in Chapter 9). You are smart, you are going to study a highly competitive course at university, so show your range of vocabulary.

### 7: Using "one" instead of "I" and "my"

This sounds pretentious. "I" and "my" are much more engaging.

*Example -- not so good:*

"Work experience abroad is essential for improving one's understanding of how different cultural attitudes towards animals are."

*Example -- better:*

"Visiting an abattoir in Oman, through family contacts, highlighted the cultural nature of attitudes towards animals, and that being aware of and sensitive towards these is essential to being a good vet."

**8: Subject abuse**

Frequent use of "I" at the start of a sentence can make you sound big-headed (and repetitive).

e.g. "I gained" / "I developed" / "I learnt" / "I joined" / "I took part in" / "I lead"

Using gerunds (a verb plus "ing") at the start of sentences is psychologically more active, saves characters, and, most importantly, gives that bounce and enthusiasm that admission tutors are looking for in a Personal Statement.

*Example -- better:*

“The way in which religion can influence people’s view of medical ethics, especially on contentious issues such as abortion and euthanasia, was something I learned first-hand when leading the school’s Ethics Society. This is an aspect of Nursing I would like to learn more about at university level.”

### 9. Being overly chatty

Your Personal Statement is a piece of serious academic writing, not a Facebook message to a friend.

*Example -- not so good:*

“My Aunt Lisa, who has worked in hospitals most of her life ... ”

*Example -- better:*

“Discussing NHS management challenges with relatives who have worked in the medical field for many years ...”

### 10: Exclamation marks

Just do not use them. Not one! Certainly not more!!!

## 11: Abbreviations

Whether referring to a school society or an aspect of biology, what you are writing about may be obvious to you but not to admissions tutors.

*Example -- not so good:*

"Taking part in the USBC summer school / Whitgift SNAP has developed ..."

*Example -- better:*

"Taking part in a local charity (Whitgift SNAP) involved organising a summer fair with a group of volunteers and developed my communication skills and rapport-building."

## 12: Starting a sentence with "And"

This is a stylistic preference rather than a grammatical rule. Though not wrong as such, the expression is best left in fiction writing where you might be aiming for dramatic effect, not in your Personal Statement.

*Example -- not so good:*

"<u>And</u>, listening to Jeremy Hunt's announcement on Radio 4 that he would put greater pressure on NHS trusts to avoid medical mistakes underlined the constant interplay between politics and medical practice in the UK."

*Example -- better:*

"Jeremy Hunt's speech regarding the decisions to put pressure on NHS trusts to avoid medical mistakes served to further emphasise how medical practice can be influenced by the current political agenda."

### 13: Starting a sentence with "But"

As above, this is not grammatically incorrect, but many people do not like it (especially English teachers and admissions tutors). The additional risk in using this construction is that it creates a sense of surprise you probably did not intend to convey.

*Example -- not so good:*

"I was sceptical about the positive impact of placebos. But, seeing my friend feel noticeably calmer before exams when taking homeopathic pills for stress made me realise how significant and positive the physical changes of this psychological boost can be."

*Example -- better:*

"My initial scepticism of placebos, despite reading a BMJ article by [XYZ] about how they could and should be prescribed to positive effect, was allayed when seeing first-hand how my friend's pre-exam nerves were significantly calmed by taking homeopathic pills."

**BANNED WORDS**

### 1: "to be able"

This is a waste of characters. The examples below show why.

*Example -- not so good:*

"By completing the Duke of Edinburgh's Gold Award I was able to improve my communication skills and ability to organise myself."

*Examples -- better:*

"By completing the Duke of Edinburgh's Gold Award I improved my communication skills and ability to organise myself."

"My communication and organisational skills, both vital for degree-level study, have been significantly improved by completing the Duke of Edinburgh's Gold Award."

### 2: "had to"

Another way to waste characters; compare the examples below.

*Example -- not so good:*

"Running the Biology Society at school meant <u>I had to organise</u> several guest speakers and motivate students to give short talks. "

*Example -- better:*

"Running the Biology Society at school meant <u>organising</u> several guest speakers and motivating students to give short talks."

### 3: "relish"

Relish belongs on burgers - with cheese.

*Example - not so good:*

"I would <u>relish</u> the opportunity to study Medicine at degree level."

*Example -- better:*

"Studying Medicine for the next five years is what I want to do because it enables me to study [XYZ] in detail, gain clinical experience, and then ultimately pursue a career as a virologist."

### 4: "thrive"

Write this about plants growing in your back garden, not about yourself at university. Prove that university will be the right place for you by giving evidence instead.

*Example -- not so good:*

"I thrive on hard work."

*Examples -- better:*

"Self-studying an extra AS-level demonstrates my willingness to commit to do what is necessary to achieve my goals." (Giving an example of how you thrive on hard work)

"Choosing to do an EPQ in addition to four A-levels evidences my ability to prioritise and meet multiple deadlines, which will be useful skills at university." (As above)

### 5: "passion" and "desire"

Neither of these words proves your interest in your subject. Let me say it again: expressions like this are empty - only specific examples show that you are passionate about your subject.

*Examples -- not so good:*

"My passion for Chemistry confirms I want to do this as a degree and in my future career."

"My desire to study Medicine springs from a childhood incident when I had to spend ten weeks in hospital ..."

*Examples -- better:*

"I have researched the intensity of study in this Veterinary Medicine course through talking to current students at open days, family, friends, and staff at vet practices. The idea of putting theory into practice on a daily basis is one of the main draws of this degree and to a career in this field."

"Ten weeks in hospital at a young age gave me my first understanding of multidisciplinary teamwork in Medicine."

### 6: "also" and "too"

This is a Personal Statement, not a shopping list. Chapter 7 tells you in detail how to present your many extracurricular activities without falling into the "also" trap.

*Example -- not so good:*

"I am a Prefect at my school and also on the football, rugby, and cricket teams. I am active in several local charities too."

*Example -- better:*

"Combining the responsibilities of a Prefect and playing on multiple sports teams has proven my ability to effectively prioritise and plan my time, both of which are vital for successful study at university level."

### 7: "In addition" or "Additionally" at the start of a sentence

Another shopping list trap.

*Example -- not so good:*

"In addition, I play county-level netball and I am captain of the school hockey team."

*Example -- better:*

"Playing county-level netball and captaining the school hockey team have developed teamwork skills which will help with the group projects required in this degree."

## 8: “However” or “Moreover” at the start of a sentence

Again, neither is grammatically incorrect (though many people believe them to be). You probably use one or both all the time in your school essays. Correct or not, these formulations are clumsy and use up unnecessary character count. My advice is to avoid.

*Example -- not so good:*

“However, when we look at Carr's “What is History”...”

*Examples -- better:*

“Looking at Carr's “What is History” ... ”

“Carr's “What is History” shows us that ... ”

## 9: “lucky enough”

This is too informal and adds nothing to enhance the meaning of the sentence.

*Example -- not so good:*

“I was lucky enough to gain work experience with a Senior Consultant at [XY] Hospital and observed several cases including [XYZ].”

(This gives the impression that your mother / father / uncle works at the hospital and either arranged your work experience for you or is actually the Senior Consultant.)

*Example -- better:*

"Researching the causes, symptoms, and treatments for [XYZ] resulted from observing a patient with this condition during my work experience with a Senior Consultant at [XY] Hospital."

**10: "really"**

Sentences with "really" use extra words to describe rather than demonstrate. Using creative ways to emphasise something you feel or think intensely will better show your ability to write well.

*Examples -- not so good:*

"I want to study Mathematics at university because I really enjoy it."

"I get really involved in activities at school, especially in science."

"I have really, really pushed myself to understand more about animal welfare in intensive farming."

*Examples -- better:*

"What I enjoy about studying Mathematics is breaking problems into logical steps."

"Doing Biology at school has taught me the importance of accuracy and attention to detail when doing fieldwork."

"Wanting to understand more about animal welfare in intensive farming prompted me to read two papers by Defra."

### 11: "in order to"

Another clumsy formulation which uses up precious characters. With the help of the examples below, find a way to rephrase your thoughts more economically.

*Example -- not so good:*

"I have taken Additional Mathematics <u>in order to</u> make the statistical modelling papers in the first two years of the degree easier to handle."

*Example -- better:*

"Taking Additional Mathematics as an extra A-level was a conscious choice to make the statistical modelling papers in the first two years of the degree easier."

**12: "always"**

No-one has always loved a particular academic subject. Writing this does not prove your aptitude for the subject, nor does it give evidence of how you have proactively pursued your interest beyond your academic work. Prove your interest with detailed examples instead.

*Example -- not so good:*

"I have always loved taking care of people."

*Example -- better:*

"Learning about the role in the wider community for nurses in the Sociological Perspectives unit of the Health and Social Care BTEC spurred me to organise a work shadowing placement with a local district nurse."

## Chapter 4

# Personal Statement Paragraph 1: WHY THIS COURSE?

It is time to turn theory into practice and start putting your ideas down on paper. By the end of this chapter you will know what you are going to write in Paragraph 1 - the all important opener to your Personal Statement - and have a first draft of this section.

In your first paragraph you will tell the admissions tutors exactly why you want to study your chosen subject. If you are not yet clear on why, the ideas below will serve as a prompt. If you do already know, these examples will help you formulate your own reason(s) effectively.

Simply stating the reason(s) for your interest is not enough; you must find evidence to prove it. The more <u>personal</u> your statement, the more convincing it will be. That means my suggestions should be a stimulus for some deep thought and reflection before you start writing.

## FIVE SUGGESTED REASONS

### Reason 1 and 2: You love it and want to study it in more depth

There are two aspects to this statement and you must make sure you address both. Firstly, you are saying that you have a specific area of interest (within one of your A-levels or from extracurricular reading), which you want to find out more about at university. Secondly, you are acknowledging that to go into this specific area properly, you must first improve your elementary understanding of the subject.

Many degrees clearly specify that the first two years are designed to give you a broad general understanding of the subject. If this is true for your chosen course, be sure to reference it. Before you start, you must check:

(a) All four (or five if applying for Nursing) of your chosen universities have modules covering the specialisation you are talking about.

(b) In relation to this specialist area you have done at least two of the following:
- written on it (EPQ / competitions / blog - see Chapter 6);
- read about it (books / magazines / websites - see Chapter 5);
- attended lectures (public lectures / guest speakers at school / online TED talks or iTunesU / summer schools / taster days - see Chapter 6);
- completed relevant work experience where feasible (see Chapter 6).

**PLAGIARISM ALERT**

*Example:*

"I am looking to gain a broad understanding of [your subject] before learning in more detail about [your specialist area], which I wrote on in my EPQ and which interests me most, in the third year.

**Reason 3: Specific trigger**

This reason is often overdone by students, but when used well can be very effective. As mentioned in Chapter 3 in the "banned words" section, nobody has "always" loved their subject. There must have been something which triggered your interest. For example:

(a) a trip / visit;
(b) a teacher;
(c) a module in your AS course;
(d) a book you read;
(e) a lecture you attended / listened to (see Chapter 6);
(f) personal / family experience;
(g) a work experience placement.

Having worked out which event or experience it was, you then need to express how this acted as a catalyst for you to find out more about the subject and, at a later stage, to research what doing it at degree level would entail. See the examples at the end of this chapter.

## Reason 4: You are good at it

People are usually good at subjects they like and like subjects they are good at. This is a perfectly adequate reason for wanting to study a subject at university. The key is introducing evidence to prove this, rather than just stating it as fact. Talking about GCSE grades will not be enough.

## Reason 5: Career

Medicine, Dentistry, Veterinary Medicine, and Nursing are clearly vocational degrees.They provide the necessary academic training to enable you to pursue your future career and this is a strong motivation to study them. As a result, admissions tutors will certainly want to see that you are committed to the career to which your degree leads - this is why work experience is so important. A more specific idea of what particular career area you hope to work in (district nursing, paediatrics, equine, hospital-based dentistry), beyond the general notion of becoming a doctor, dentist, vet, or nurse, is even better.

That said, any explicitly stated career ambition must be coupled with genuine academic interest. Excelling at university and in your career will only be possible if you are genuinely interested in the subject matter, not just the subsequent job title. So if your main reason for your degree choice is a professional one, make sure to place enough emphasis on your academic interest in parallel.

## EXAMPLES OF OPENING PARAGRAPHS

****PLAGIARISM ALERT****

Below are examples of how to express the reasons above in an opening paragraph. In each instance, I provide a range of alternatives. This is to give you a feel of how to play around with language and use a variety of vocabulary to express the same thought in different ways. Once you move on to the writing stage, aim to build on these examples to express your personal reason.

*Example - reason 1 and 2: you love it and want to study it in more depth*

"I want to learn more about the complexities of the animals at a systemic and cellular level. What I enjoy most is looking at how such knowledge and skill can be applied."

*Or:*

"It is the combination of human interaction and deep scientific knowledge that attracts me to Medicine at degree level. The PBL approach your course takes will fit my learning style, as has been confirmed by various work experiences and taster days."

*Example - reason 3: specific trigger*

“Understanding why my grandfather needed a dialysis machine, when helping him with it as a child, made me realise how little I knew about the human body and how much I wanted to find out. I will apply that experience of seeing the accuracy and care needed to apply medical treatments effectively in my future career in Nursing. Since then ... ”

*Or:*

“Having three, rugby-playing older brothers meant that my early teens involved multiple visits to A&E. Seeing the Multi-Disciplinary-Team in action, learning about triage (why we had to wait), and observing the doctors combine academic excellence with great people skills to extract specific information gave me my initial motivation to start exploring Medicine as a university subject.”

*Example - reason 4: you are good at it*

“High achievement in school exams and at the Chemistry and Biology Olympiads (two golds) led me to consider Dentistry as a potential degree subject. The EPQ I have done on [ABC] confirmed that gaining a greater understanding of how oral health influences the whole body is what I want to do next.”

*Or:*

"Gaining a coveted place on the Imperial College Medicine Summer School was a result of my academic grades and my broad extracurricular interest in science, ranging from MERS mutations to government policy on sugar in food. Building on this, I ..."

*Example - reason 5: career*

"Multiple work experiences, MedSim, taster days, and talking to medical practitioners in my community has confirmed that I want to study Medicine at university with a long-term view of becoming a GP."

*Or:*

"My ambition is to pursue a career in medical research with a particular focus on degenerative muscular diseases. Getting a 'commended' award for my essay on research pathways for multiple sclerosis from [XXX] competition gave me the confidence that I both enjoy and can excel at the academic work covered in a Medicine degree."

## Chapter 5

# Personal Statement Paragraph 2: SUBJECT-SPECIFIC FURTHER READING

The aim in paragraph 2 is to reference and discuss the relevant books you have read, beyond what you must read for A-level. Simply listing everything you have read is not good enough: you must set out to prove your interest in and aptitude for your chosen course.

To do this, you need to intelligently analyse the ideas you have read about and draw out examples to make specific points, linking these where possible to relevant work experience. This requires actually reading sections of the books; not necessarily from cover to cover ("Introductions" and "Conclusions" plus a couple of relevant chapters can go a long way), but it will take you some time.

Below are suggestions of relevant books for your subject. For each, there are specific ideas and arguments which you could draw out of the texts and weave into your Personal Statement using the quotes I give and your own words. As before, I provide multiple examples for each idea. Use these examples to help you formulate your own ideas using a wide range of vocabulary. A longer list of potential titles is in Appendix 2.

If you are just getting started with extracurricular reading, pick two titles from the list below or in Appendix 2. Go get them from the library or a local bookshop and start reading immediately. If you have already started own reading, the below will give you ideas for other books to read and show you how to work your thoughts into your statement. Remember the quality of the examples you use is far more important than the quantity of books you have read.

****PLAGIARISM ALERT****

## (a) Medicine

### BOOK 1: "The Viral Storm" by Nathan Wolfe

<u>Idea 1: Viruses remain a relatively unknown quantity to scientists, so researching them presents an opportunity to expand human knowledge</u>

*Quote from book:*

"Viruses evolve more rapidly than any organism on the planet, yet we understand less about them than any other form of life."

*Example:*

"Just how much there is still to discover about viruses became more apparent when reading Wolfe's "The Viral Storm" and increases my fascination, " ... we understand less about them [viruses] than any other form of life." By pursuing a medical career, my ambition is to push the boundaries of medical research to help improve health globally, particularly in this vital area of research."

*Or:*

"Nathan Wolfe's research into viruses and their prevention, set out in "The Viral Storm", shows that there is still much to be done to successfully anticipate the next global pandemic. My interest in this spurred me on to organise a two-day placement shadowing with a virologist at UCL - an insight into what the virology module in the second year of this course will begin to cover."

Idea 2: The interdisciplinary approach required for viable medical research into viruses

*Quote from book:*

"... we no longer live on a planet where pockets of life persist for centuries without contact with others. We now live on a microbially unified planet."

*Example:*

"Reading Wolfe's "The Viral Storm" on our "microbially unified planet" emphasised that medical research can only be successful if produced and analysed in the context of other research disciplines. This is especially true in virology, in which an understanding of global movements and future ways in which people will organise their lives is essential - for which my Sociology A-Level prepares me well."

*Or:*

"When researching my EPQ on "Anticipating the Next Pandemic" I included sociology and geography articles on current and future migration patterns. Accurately modelling these aspects of globalisation is crucial to creating an accurate picture of our "microbially unified planet" (Wolfe - "The Viral Storm) and further virology research."

**BOOK 2: "The Shape We're In" by Sarah Boseley**

<u>Idea 1: Identifying the root of health problems involves looking at the patient's lifestyle and building a rapport with the patient so that he or she is willing to share these details and to listen to what the doctor recommends.</u>

*Quote from book:*

"James admits he is probably in a minority of GPs in speaking to his patients about their weight when they come in for other reasons, such as problems with their knees or their feet."

*Example:*

"The labelling of my hometown, Tamworth, as the "fattest town in Britain" motivated my interest in doctor / patient collaboration to reverse the growing obesity crisis. Boswell's observation in "The Shape We're In" that few GPs "speak to patients about their weight when they come in for other reasons, such as problems with their knees or feet", emphasised how a patient presenting with a specific complaint is an opportunity for doctors to improve patients' lifestyles and overall health. Developing clinical skills which allow me to do this is one essential aspect of what I hope to achieve during this medical degree."

*Or:*

"Based on my work experience, I hope to become a GP because of the opportunity it presents to positively impact of patients' lifestyles as a way of preventing more serious future medical complications. Reading Boswell's "The Shape We're In" highlighted that simply investing a little time in building rapport with a patient so as to talk to them honestly about their weight can avoid years of expensive treatment later in life."

<u>Idea 2: Doctors' role in shaping public health policy.</u>

*Quote from book:*

"The UK's public health doctors are on board ... In an important statement, she [Lindsey Davies, president of the Faculty of Public Health] backed the call for cross-departmental action from the government - and slammed politicians for blaming people for their weight."

*Example:*

"I am interested in the correlation between legislating against tobacco and, in the future, against sugar. As in the 1960s, medical opinion on the obesity epidemic in Britain is becoming increasingly politicised. As Boswell writes in "The Shape We're In", working on the frontline, doctors across many disciplines - e.g. psychology, cardiology, bariatric surgery - are urging government to see obesity as more than a matter of individual responsibility and put through legislation that helps people stop consuming such large quantities of sugar."

*Or:*

"Far greater investment on a national scale, spearheaded by the medical community, will be essential for improving standards of health in Britain. The ideas in Boswell's "The Shape We're In" confirmed my view on the need for greater for legislation in the soft drinks and snack food industries; the role doctors play in making the public health case for this to government is one of my motivations for studying this course."

### (b) Dentistry

**BOOK 1: “Bad Science” by Ben Goldacre**

Idea 1: The use of ‘noble myths’ (complicated-sounding scientific justifications) in dental care as a way of motivating patients to follow dentist’s advice.

*Quote from book:*

“ ... you can use hocus pocus - or what Plato euphemistically called a ‘noble myth’ - to make people do something fairly sensible like drink some water and have an exercise break.”

*Example:*

“Having read Ben Goldacre’s reference to “noble myths” in “Bad Science” I started considering the ways in which a dentist might present simple common-sense ideas about general health as a way of improving dental health without medical intervention - such as not letting small children suck their thumbs for too long.”

*Or:*

“Following a two-week placement at a local children’s dental practice and having read Ben Goldacre’s “Bad Science”, I now appreciate how placebos can actually play a positive role in health and dental care. Even something non-medical, such as giving children a fun sticker with the promise that it will help them feel better, has a powerful effect in making them believe that."

Idea 2: Producing effective and accurate research based on systematic reviews, as opposed to contorting selective evidence to fit with your desired argument.

*Quote from book:*

"Systematic reviews are one of the great ideas of modern thought. They should be celebrated."

*Example:*

"As a scientist, I strive for accuracy in my work, but it was first on reading Goldacre's scathing attack of the methods used in many studies in "Bad Science" that alerted me to how inaccurate conclusions presented as truths often are. Noting Goldacre's emphasis on the value of systematic reviews, I broadened my research for my EPQ on the addition of fluoride in drinking water to include a better spectrum of studies, despite their conclusions not always supporting the point I wanted to make."

*Or:*

"Goldacre's suggestion in "Bad Science" that many scientific studies are inaccurate in their conclusions - manipulating results to fit with the argument the scientist is trying to make and ignoring outlying data - has encouraged me to become more critical when reading scientific journals, such as XYZ, and science articles in broadsheet newspapers. This ability to question what I read will be much needed for university study."

**BOOK 2: "The Complete Pre-Dental Guide to Modern Dentistry" by John Syrbu**

<u>Idea 1: The level of detailed scientific knowledge required at degree-level and beyond.</u>

*Quote from book:*

"The practice of oral pathology includes research and diagnosis of diseases using clinical, radiographic, microscopic, biochemical, or other examinations."

*Example:*

"With its focus on microscopic and biochemical examinations, my long-term career goal is to specialise in oral pathology, which I learned more about from Syrbu's "Complete Pre-Dental Guide to Modern Dentistry".

*Or:*

"The high-level scientific scope of Dentistry, both at degree-level and as a practising dentist, as shown in Syrbu's "Complete Pre-

Dental Guide to Modern Dentistry", is exciting, especially in oral pathology; the area in which I later aim to specialise."

Idea 2: Dentistry is both an art and science in that teeth problems can cause both functional and aesthetic problems.

*Quote from book:*

"Spacing and crowding are common in the human dentition but may cause both esthetic and functional problems."

*Example:*

"For patients, aesthetics are often the motivating factor when straightening teeth. Reading Syrbu's "Complete Pre-Dental Guide to Modern Dentistry" emphasised the perhaps more pressing "functional problems", such as an increased caries risk, that can arise if teeth are either too small for their arch or overcrowded because of a discrepancy between tooth size and room available in the dental arch. My work experience at a paediatric dental practice confirmed this."

*Or:*

"Having observed a paediatric dentist, I realised that the best way to encourage adolescents to accept wearing a brace to correct either overcrowding or spacing (if teeth are too small for their arch) is not to emphasise the "functional problems" (as highlighted in Syrbu's

"The Complete Pre-Dental Guide to Modern Dentistry"), but to explain how the long-term aesthetic of their teeth will be improved - a more immediate concern for most 14-year-olds than an increased risk of caries."

### (c) Veterinary Science

**BOOK 1: "Life at the Extremes" by Frances Ashcroft**

<u>Idea 1: Vets' educative role in preventative care and animal welfare.</u>

*Quote from book:*

"Closer to home, dogs hang their moist tongues out of their mouths to accelerate heat loss and pant to cause cooling of the nasal passages and facilitate evaporative heat loss from the upper airways."

*Example:*

"Learning about how mammals respond to extreme heat in Ashcroft's "Life at the Extremes" prompted me to think about the crucial role vets play in educating pet owners on the symptoms of overexposure. A dog's welfare is significantly increased (and illnesses are prevented) if an owner can respond quickly and appropriately to panting, tongue hanging out, for example, by simply providing rest, shade, and water."

*Or:*

"Being an observant pet owner is key to maintaining good animal health. From providing balanced nutrition and vigorous exercise, to understanding how an animal's body might react in extreme conditions (a dog panting, tongue hanging out when overheated, for example - per Ashcroft's "Life at the Extremes"), the opportunity vets have to promote sensitivity to animals' needs is one reason why I am committed to a career in small animal practice."

<u>Idea 2: The breadth of animal biology and wider applications of this set of scientific knowledge.</u>

*Quote from book:*

"Animals also adapt to chronic cold by biochemical changes within their cells that enables them to operate at lower temperatures."

*Example:*

"I am interested in how animals adapt to their environment at a biochemical level, per Ashcroft in "Life at the Extremes" on the nature of fats in cell membranes. This shows the breadth of biochemical understanding required by vets for ensuring animal welfare, as well as how this knowledge can aid advancements in human medicine."

*Or:*

"The traditional, domestic application of animal products - using neat's foot oil to soften leather, for example (per Ashcroft's "Life at the Extremes") - can reveal much about animals' biochemical adaptation to their environment. Coupled with modern and detailed scientific research, such observations can be used effectively to create ideal living conditions for animals, even if reared for farming.

**BOOK 2: "The Viral Storm" by Nathan Wolfe**

<u>Idea 1: The taxonomic transmission rule.</u>

*Quote from book:*

"The idea is that the more closely related any two species are, the higher the probability that a microbe can successfully jump between them." (Dogs and wolves, humans and chimpanzees)

*Example:*

"Zoobiquity" by Horowitz and Bowers has helped me understand my current affairs reading on the MERS virus with its likely origins in cave bats, infecting camels, and then jumping to humans. All three being mammals is significant in the successful transfer of the virus. This is even more likely in more physiologically similar animals (e.g. dogs and wolves, humans and chimpanzees), per Wolfe's taxonomic transmission rule "the more closely related any two species are, the higher the probability that a microbe can successfully jump between them" in "The Viral Storm".

*Or:*

"The recent poultry industry crisis, uncovered by the Guardian in July, highlights just one aspect of how vets work to improve public health. According to the Federation of Veterinarians of Europe, 75% of emerging diseases are zoonoses (diseases transmissible between animal and man). Understanding the pathologies and stages of transmission (between different types of animals), including the likelihood of transmission using Wolfe's "taxonomic transmission rule" ("The Viral Storm"), is another important way in which vets can improve both animal and human health - an area I look forward to learning more about in this course."

<u>Idea 2: Studying the interaction of domestic and wild animals gives one of the main clues to the origins of new viruses in farm animals and humans.</u>

*Quote from book:*

"... the threat from domestic animals comes more from them acting as bridges to allow the movement of wild animal microbes into the human population. ... Clearly, when it comes to new pandemics, wild animals are where the action is."

*Example:*

"Prohibiting dog walking on farmland during the 2007 foot and mouth crisis was just one example of the role of vets in public health issues - as outlined in Wolfe's "threat from domestic animals comes more from them acting as bridges [for viruses]" in "The Viral Storm".

*Or:*

"The essential role vets play in identifying and preventing the transmission of viruses (such as rabies) between wild animals, domestic animals ("acting as bridges" per Wolfe's "The Viral Storm"), and ultimately humans shows the potential in this career to influence both public and animal health."

### (d) Nursing

### BOOK 1: "The Spirit Catches You and You Fall Down" by Anne Fadiman

Idea 1: Dual role of nurses in administering medical care and supporting families in administering this care to relatives / children.

*Quote from book:*

"By the time she was four and half, Lia's parents had been told to give her, at various times, Tylemol, ampicillin, amoxicillin, Dilantin, phenobarbital, erythromycin, Ceclor, Tegretol, Benadryl, Pediazole, Vi-Daylin Multivitamins with Iron, Alupent, Depakene, and Valium."

*Example:*

"The complex drug regime (Dilantin, phenobarbital, Tegretol, plus antibiotics and vitamins) given to a young child to control serious epilepsy in Fadiman's "The Spirit Catches You and You Fall Down" highlighted both the challenge in combining medicines to achieve the best patient outcome, as well as in communicating this effectively to the family who must administer them, often without understanding each drug's purpose. Nurses play an essential role in observing how the patient reacts to various drugs, and supporting families in caring for their sick relative."

*Or:*

"My younger brother has epilepsy, so I was especially drawn to Fadiman's "The Spirt Catches You and You Fall Down". Reading how the family were overwhelmed and confused by the complex drug regime their epileptic daughter required (Dilantin, phenobarbital, Tegretol, amongst others) showed me how essential the excellent nursing care my brother has received is in helping him control his condition. The opportunity to support families by providing ongoing care in the community has motivated my career choice."

<u>Idea 2: Nurses need to be sensitive to cultural differences to treat patients without causing any distress.</u>

*Quote from book:*

"Do American doctors eat the livers, kidneys, and brains of Hmong patients? ... The limited contact the Hmong had already had with Western medicine in the camp hospitals and clinics had done little to instill confidence, ..."

*Example:*

"I have a special interest in the current Ebola epidemic in West Africa, as my family is originally from Sierra Leone and we still have relatives living in the region. From articles I have read in the Guardian and on the BBC, it seems clear to me that much of what is hindering the containment of the epidemic are local suspicions of Western medicine. This linked up with what I had read in "The Spirit Catches You and You Fall Down" by Anne Fadiman, and underlines the importance of culturally sensitive nursing and medical practice, especially in communities with large numbers of recent immigrants."

*Or:*

"Given the financial constraints within the NHS, I used to question the value of additional services such as providing a translator. Reading "The Spirit Catches You and You Fall Down" by Anne Fadiman (recommended to me by the district nurse I shadowed for two weeks) opened my eyes to the importance of medical staff being able to effectively communicate with patients, so as to accurately diagnose, treat, instil confidence, and avoid frightening misconceptions, such as Western "doctors each livers". A translator's fee is a small price to pay."

**BOOK 2: "Call the Midwife" by Jennifer Worth**

<u>Idea 1: Effective community nursing involves looking at the patient's circumstances in order to give the best advice.</u>

*Quote from book:*

"As I glanced around the crowded room, the minimal kitchen area, and the general lack of facilities, it flashed through my mind that bottle-feeding would be the worst thing for the baby."

*Example:*

"Reading "Call the Midwife" inspired me to set up a work shadowing placement with a local district nurse. Even today, nurses visiting people's homes is essential for gaining an in-depth understanding of how best to care for patients, just as it was 60 years ago when Jennifer Worth glanced around her patient's room to see "bottle-feeding would be the worst thing for the baby."

*Or:*

"I am keen to pursue district nursing as a future career. Jennifer Worth's books on nursing and midwifery in the East End of London in the 1950s, which I read for fun, helped spur my interest. Her vivid observations illustrated to me how a good nurse must want to understand patients on a personal level, including their home environment - which ties in with my A-levels in Psychology and Sociology.

<u>Idea 2: Creating a feeling of trust with a patient and understanding that different patients respond to different methods of communication are the first steps to providing good nursing care.</u>

*Quote from book:*

"From that moment on, Mrs Jenkins lost her fear of us. We were able to examine her, to treat her, to communicate with her."

*Example:*

"The scene in Worth's "Call the Midwife", when one of the nuns uses an unusual method to gain the trust of a frightened old lady showed me that gentle humour can be a great way of helping set aside a patient's anxiety. This is especially true with children, as I discovered during work experience on the Children's Ward at my local hospital. I found that making a fun game of putting on the oxygen mask helped many children stay calm."

*Or:*

"Establishing patient trust can be hard, even for skilled and experienced nurses, as I realised when reading "Call the Midwife" by Jennifer Worth. Her description of how the nuns used humour to connect with frightened patients so that they could "examine, treat and communicate" with them has already helped improve my approach with the elderly people I care for at weekends in a nearby care home."

## Chapter 6

# Personal Statement Paragraph 3: SUBJECT-SPECIFIC EXTRACURRICULAR ACTIVITIES

When applying for highly competitive, vocational courses, such as Medicine, Dentistry, Veterinary Medicine, and Nursing, it is absolutely essential to complete relevant work experience and voluntary work, and then weave your reflections on these experiences into your statement. Indeed, many universities state explicitly on course websites the minimum amount of relevant work experience they expect you to have completed before application.

Whether this is the case for your course or not, all admissions tutors want to see relevant work experience to show that you understand the day-to-day reality of your chosen profession and that you have proven your commitment to it, above and beyond other potential candidates.

As with all of your preparation for your Personal Statement, how you present what you have done is crucial. A list of placements will not do. You must show admissions tutors that you have reacted intelligently to placements and learned from them, referencing them as the trigger for reading a particular book in paragraph 2 or detailing an opinion you formed as a result of this experience, plus further reading or an online lecture, in paragraph 3.

Work experience and voluntary work remain paramount, but you might want to make brief reference to a few additional activities related to your subject. The options beyond work experience are many: watching / attending lectures; regularly reading (and that means not just subscribing to!) a relevant magazine; joining a society at school - to name just a few.

Much of what you can do, watch, or read is available online, which means access to London is not required. Again, quality is more important than quantity. If you are just starting out, pick two work experience placements, plus three or four different lectures / activities, complete them, and then bring these into your statement. That is plenty.

If you are already involved in one or more of the below, the examples will show you how to link your current activities with your other thoughts on your subject and provide ideas for further activities, if you have time.

****PLAGIARISM ALERT****

## 1. Work Experience

Arranging placements requires initiative. Unless you are exceptionally lucky and well-connected, these will not fall into your lap. Other candidates will be arranging these for themselves; to beat the competition, you must as well. Pick an area which interests you, get on the phone, find out who to email, and organise it for yourself.

Taking the initiative to gain more experience in a particular area is exactly the sort of motivation that impresses admissions tutors, so do include details on how the placement came about. Aim for two-week placements, or two separate, one-week placements in different practices / hospital departments.

### (a) Medicine

i) GP work shadowing
ii) Local health clinic
iii) Local hospital
iv) Specialist unit in local hospital, either inpatient or outpatient (good to have experience of both)
v) Visiting a clinic or doctor's surgery in another country (if you have the language skills and contacts)

*Example:*

"Encountering the complexity of opportunistic cancers in HIV clinics while observing the MDT of the Oncology Department at St James Hospital (Newcastle) showed me how diverse even a specialised area of Medicine can be and the reality of "life-long learning". Discussing cell signalling in more detail on the wards with [XX] led me to read Leroi's "Mutants" and subsequently research the most frequently disrupted pathways when cancers are present, such as IGF."

### (b) Dentistry

i) General dentist practice
ii) Orthodontist
iii) Radiography department at local hospital
iv) Dental laboratory
v) Oral and maxillofacial surgery
vi) Community Dental Practice

*Example:*

"To ensure I make the strongest application possible, my approach to preparing for it has been methodical. This has involved organising a range of work experience placements, through school contacts, family friends, and cold calling. Three days in the Radiography Department of my local hospital was the result of six emails, two phone calls, and an informal interview. The time there was hugely informative about how to "read" and "interpret" X-rays. As a result of this contact I was introduced to a maxillofacial surgeon and will have a week of shadowing and observation next summer."

### (c) Veterinary Medicine

i) Local veterinary practice
ii) Local farm
iii) Placement in an abattoir
iv) Placement in a local zoo

*Example:*

"Treating equine sarcoids with the human BCG vaccine reinforced the complexity of inter-species infection and cure. Working alongside standard treatments with a specialist equine vet at a racehorse yard in Sussex, I was intrigued when told that the trainer would bring in a holistic Reiki healer to speed up the recovery process of a foreleg fracture."

**(d) Nursing**

i) Local health clinic
ii) Local hospital
iii) Specialist unit in local hospital, either inpatient or outpatient (good to have experience of both)
iv) Residential care home for the elderly
v) Visiting a clinic or doctor's surgery in another country (if you have the language skills and contacts)

*Example:*

"To help me identify the area which suited me best, I organised a number of work experience placements. Since then, twelve months volunteering in both a residential home for the elderly and an under-5s playgroup have provided an invaluable insight into the patience and communication skills required when dealing with either group, but it was with the children that I felt most comfortable."

## 2. Volunteering

### (a) Medicine

i) Residential home for the elderly
ii) Activities with children in hospital / hospice
iii) St John's Ambulance

*Example:*

"For the last three years, I have been a member of St John's Ambulance. Using the skills taught twice - both while volunteering at my local football stadium - has increased my determination to study Medicine. In the first instance a man had an epileptic fit and, in the second, a child fainted (as a result of heat and dehydration). In both cases I responded quickly and provided first aid until the paramedics arrived."

### (b) Dentistry

i) Residential home for the elderly
ii) Local hospital
iii) Dental nurse school visits

*Example:*
"Wanting to understand more about dentistry and public health, I volunteered for two months with a local dental practice, accompanying a dental nurse on trips to primary schools and

nurseries. The purpose of these visits (once a week, coinciding with a free morning in school) is to explain to children the importance of good dental hygiene. Having observed the dental nurse twice, I became the main presenter; an excellent way to learn how approachable you need to be when treating children."

### (c) Veterinary Medicine

i) Relevant charity (RSPCA, PSPCB, local animal rescue)
ii) Local kennels
iii) Animal sanctuary

*Example:*

"I started volunteering at a local rescue shelter for cats and dogs, having seen how vets must be able to deal well with distressed animals during my work experience. Hands-on experience caring for the animals that come in (often with a history of abuse) has been challenging but vital in understanding how to slowly build up an animal's trust and calm them down."

### (d) Nursing

i) See three Medicine examples above
ii) Local nursery
iii) Community centre / youth club

*Example:*

"Helping disabled teenagers get dressed in the mornings has been one of the responsibilities in my voluntary role at a local respite centre. Many patients had very particular ideas on what they wanted to wear and how they wanted me to help them. From this, I learned that patience and sense of humour go a long way in easing potentially sensitive or embarrassing situations."

## 3. Free Lectures

### (a) Medicine

i) Royal College of Surgeons: *http://www.rcseng.ac.uk/museums/hunterian/events/audio-video-and-transcripts*

The RCS organises regular lunchtime and evening lectures on a host of relevant medical topics. Events are ticketed, but inexpensive (£4 per person). Past lectures can be downloaded on the website, either as an audio, transcript, or video.

*Example:*

"The Christmas Lecture at the Royal College of Surgeons on the benefits of laparoscopic surgery underlined the way medical professionals need to be adaptable and prepared for life-long learning. The changes witnessed over 40 years by a doctor retiring in 2014, including the introduction of complex technology, the eradication of polio, and the emergence of new killers such as AIDS, emphasise how doctors experience and drive major societal change - and this is what I want."

ii) Institute of Psychiatry (King's College London): *http://www.kcl.ac.uk/ioppn/news/engagement/index.aspx*

The IoP runs a range of day-long events, some available to students. Another idea is to attend or listen to a Maudsley Debate - arranged three times a year and open to the public. Speakers are prominent medical practitioners and other public figures; topics focus on current points of contention in mental health and mental healthcare. Podcasts of past debates are available for download on the website.

*Example:*

"Accessing the Alzheimer's Day at the Institute of Psychiatry, as part of the Kings College K+ programme, and the lab tour and talks on current strategies by scientists and doctors, gave me a much deeper understanding of this common condition. This inspired me to start a briefing sheet on the causes, symptoms, treatment, and recent discoveries for the most life-affecting conditions in the UK, the research for which took me into more detail on the role of plaque and tangles."

iii) Royal College of Physicians: *http://www.rcplondon.ac.uk/events/public-events*

The RCP hosts a series of public events and exhibitions, providing a fascinating insight into health, medicine, and science. Talks by a diverse assortment of speakers cover the history of medicine, aspects of public health, and much more.

### (b) Dentistry

i) The Dentistry Show: *http://www.thedentistryshow.co.uk/*

This is an annual industry event for all dentists, practice managers, dental hygienists, therapists, and nurses. It serves as an opportunity for companies to display latest technological advancements, as well as a forum to discuss recent developments in dentistry. Under-18s are not permitted to attend, but some videos of lectures and talks at past events are available online.

*Example:*

"Watching online a talk by "Heart Your Smile" at the Dentistry Show gave me a good understanding of how the industry is pushing to improve its public perception and gain public trust."

ii) British Dental Association / Lindsay Society History of Dentistry: *http://www.bda.org/museum/dental-links/lindsay/*

Part of the BDA, the Lindsay Society was set up in 1962 to honour the history of dentistry. Named after Lilian Lindsay, the first female to qualify as a dentist in the UK, it runs yearly lectures on topics such as the role of dentists in society and how treatment has changed through the ages.

*Example:*

"I am interested in the history of dentistry, and independently arranged to attend the Lindsay Society's annual memorial lecture on the history of dentistry in the UK Armed Forces. The importance of easy access to dental care during conflict and peace served to underline the wider societal role of dentists."

iii) The John McLean Archive: *http://mcleanarchive.bda.org/history/default.aspx*

An online resource containing the transcripts (and some recordings) of oral histories of prominent dentists, this website will help you discover a breadth of dentistry experiences, from long-standing general practitioners who went on to influence public policy, to hygienists talking about the changing attitudes towards their work.

**(c) Veterinary Medicine**

i) Royal Veterinary College School Tour: *http://www.rvc.ac.uk/Undergraduate/VisitUs/RVCOnTour/index.cfm*

Each September the RVC holds events across the country for prospective students and parents. Free to attend, these are a great opportunity to find out more about studying this course and the career paths available in the veterinary field.

*Example:*

"Using my own research and organisational initiative, I arranged to attend and travel to the the RVC event in Birmingham. Talking to current students about the balance between practical and classroom learning confirmed that this course will suit my hands-on nature and provide a deep scientific foundation for future specialisation in my particular area of interest - reproduction and herd in farm animal medicine."

ii) Grant Museum of Zoology (UCL): *http://www.ucl.ac.uk/museums/zoology/whats-on*

Housing London's leading collection of animal specimens, the Grant Museum was originally set up as a teaching museum, but is now very much a public institution, With around 67,000 specimens, some of which are from now extinct animals, it represents a great resource for prospective students of Veterinary Medicine. They hold a number of lectures and events throughout the year, which are free to attend, and cover topics, such as "Animals and Engineering"; "Explore Zoology", and country-specific animal explorations.

## (d) Nursing

i) Charities, such as MIND: *www.mind.org.uk/*

Some health charities, such as MIND, organise lectures on wider social topics. These can be great places to find out more from an expert about a particular area of interest, in an informal, extracurricular setting.

*Example:*

"Common mental health disorders are one of my areas of interest. To improve my understanding, I have been seeking out lectures and presentations given by charities to widen the public's understanding. A recent example was a MIND lecture on Asberger's Syndrome. Having read "The Curious Incident of the Dog in the Nighttime" I thought I knew what to expect, but the sheer talent of many people with Asberger's and the way the condition can strengthen abilities, such as focus and attention to detail, was revealing."

ii) Local NHS centres

Some local NHS centres organise support groups or talks to help educate the public on a particular aspect of health. Look up your local centres, and ask them whether they have anything relevant coming up, which you might be able to attend as a prospective Nursing student.

*Example:*

"I found out about a talk at a local support group for young mothers and asked the organisers if I would be able to attend, because I wanted to know more about community nursing. They agreed, after first checking with the attendees. Attending gave me a good insight into the physical, emotional, and financial struggles this group face."

### 4. TED Talks, iTunesU, US Universities

Without a doubt, these three are the greatest resource on the web for Personal Statement material. The videos are usually only 15 - 20 minutes long and include thousands of topics under specific headings discussed by world leaders in their subject. As with other lectures, the trick is not to describe what you watched but to engage with the ideas, to give an opinion, and to link to other extracurricular or school material.

i) TED talks: *https://www.ted.com/talks*
ii) iTunesU: *http://www.apple.com/education/ipad/itunes-u/*
iii) US universities: *Harvard*, *Stamford*, *Yale*, *Berkley*, *Columbia*

#### (a) Medicine

*http://www.ted.com/talks/stephen_friend_the_hunt_for_unexpected_genetic_heroes*

*Example:*

"I believe Stephen Friend's unexpected genetic heroes idea, which suggests that preventative genetic research involves studying those who do not get sick despite carrying genes for a particular condition, is the way forward. Looking at what blocks coronary disease exhibiting, despite a patient having excessive lipid levels, emphasises the exciting prospects in medical research and is a major reason why I want to study this degree."

*Or:*

*http://www.ted.com/talks/tristram_wyatt_the_smelly_mystery_of_the_human_pheromone*

"Tristram Wyatt's TED lecture on pheromones, and in particular the background story on how half a million silk moths were used by a German scientific team after twenty years of research to identify the first pheromone molecules, exemplifies the qualities needed in the medical field. I believe I have the academic ability, patience, logic, and creativity to succeed in diagnosis and care-based decision-making."

**(b) Dentistry**

See examples above for Medicine.

## (c) Veterinary Medicine

i) See examples above for Medicine.

ii) *http://www.ted.com/talks/ ian_dunbar_on_dog_friendly_dog_training*

*Example:*

“Ian Dunbar’s TED talk on how effective dog training must take the dog’s perspective into account resonated with my direct experience volunteering in a local kennels. It is unfair and unrealistic to expect an animal to respond to human commands that it has not yet learned. To understand more about the emotional intelligence required to care for animals I have arranged to shadow a dog trainer for two weeks in the autumn half term.”

## (d) Nursing

*http://www.ted.com/talks/ eric_dishman_take_health_care_off_the_mainframe*

*Example:*

“Dishman's “take healthcare off the mainframe” TED talk reinforced my own experience of working with the elderly in care homes. The day-to-day observations that care staff and nurses cam make and the behavioural patterns they can track are essential in identifying early indicators to healthcare problems. The fact that an elderly person is gradually taking longer to reach the 'recognition moment' of who they are speaking to on the phone or the ongoing quiet ending of a voice over an extended period can point towards Alzheimer's or Parkinson's. This people-based observation and care network is what I want to be a part of.

## 5. Competitions

Taking part in competitions (even if you do not win) shows you in a good light in several ways. You had the initiative to find out that the competitions existed and then act on that information. You completed independent research and project work without (or with only minimal) support from school, which is what will be expected of you at university. To complete the trio, you did all of this on top of your current studies, which shows you can prioritise and deal with pressure.

### (a) Medicine and Veterinary Science

i) Young Scientist of the Year Award: *http://www.nsecuk.org/Get_Started/*

*Example:*

"My independent research skills and ability to motivate myself are shown by my entry for the Young Scientist of the Year Award. This involved writing an essay on sugar consumption and the potential for alternatives such as stevia, for which I was short-listed as one of 360 finalists. With the prospect of testing my lab skills against students nationally at the Big Bang Fair in March, I have been practising these in additional weekly lunchtime lab sessions."

## (b) Dentistry

i) Young Enterprise: *www.young-enterprise.org.uk/*

Long-term, many dentists may run or be a partner in a practice. To do this successfully, they need good business acumen and commercial drive. Involvement in Young Enterprise, as a student studying predominantly science subjects, is a great way of getting some useful experience and making your Personal Statement stand out.

*Example:*

"My commitment to achieving highly in the national Young Enterprise competition, as well as the standard Biology and Chemistry Olympiads (for which I gained silver and gold medals), was with a view to my future career. Running a dental practice (or a chain of them) is a commercial proposition and I wanted to understand the driving forces of business in a practical way. This is important as I study neither Business nor Economics. Persuading my group to make me leader was the first challenge overcome. Since, I have dedicated over one hundred hours of my free time to refining our product, our pitch, and building our marketing campaign. I consider having reached and won the Regional Finals a great success, as our school had never previously gone beyond local inter-school stage."

### (c) Nursing

i) The National Schools Challenge: *http://schoolschallenge.targetjobs.co.uk/*

Run by Target Jobs, this nationwide competition is a brilliant opportunity to show that you are competitive, able, and willing to put in additional hard work to stand out from your peers. Despite its business and commercial focus, the competition tests decision-making, teamwork, leadership, and creativity, all of which are highly relevant for a career in nursing.

*Example:*

"Getting through to the Grand Final of the National Schools Challenge was a huge confidence boost. Using my skills of decision-making and teamwork proved to me that, with training, I have what it takes to work in a high-pressured hospital environment as part of a multi-disciplinary team."

## 6. Taster Courses

These subject-specific university experience days are fantastic proof that you are serious about choosing the right course for you.

### (a) Medicine

i) Medsim: *http://www.workshop-uk.net/medsim*

*Example:*

"The experience of using the laparoscopic surgery simulator at Medsim was intense (in terms of concentration and precision), but emphasised that I have the fine motor skills so essential for a doctor, in part developed by fifteen years of daily violin practice."

### (b) Dentistry

i) Dentistry Workshop: *http://workshop-uk.net/dentistry-2013*

*Example:*

"Learning more about the importance of treating malocclusions for patients' physical and psychological health at the Dentistry Workshop motivated me to set up work experience with an orthodontist. Beyond aesthetics, patients reported a decrease in headaches, jaw ache, and neck problems following orthodontic treatment."

### (c) Veterinary Medicine

i) Vetsim: *http://workshop-uk.net/vetsim*

*Example:*

"To gain first-hand experience of practical procedures, not possible during work placements, was one of my main motives for attending Vetsim last year. Mastering the suturing technique was exhilarating and has given me the confidence that I have the practical skills necessary for this course."

### (d) Nursing

i) Nursing Workshop: *http://workshop-uk.net/nursing*

*Example:*

"The Nursing Workshop introduced me to the diagnostic role of nurses. Being in a hands-on, caregiving role, nurses' observations are essential in helping doctors make a preliminary diagnosis - a nursing skill I am looking forward to developing at university."

## 7. Magazines / Websites

A number highly academic and well-regarded science and medical magazines have extensive websites, where many (if not all) of their articles and latest research are published. This makes them a brilliant and essential source of cutting edge news and hot topics.

Note that most students applying for your course will say that they read this sort of publication. A brief mention in your Personal Statement that you read these publications is not enough. It is reading regularly and analysing the information you find that will give you valuable content. You must then intelligently work in these ideas to show an opinion you have formed, how you have connected these with work experience or other reading, and, of course, how all of this combines to prove your suitability for the degree.

### (a) Medicine

i) BMJ*: www.bmj.com/*
ii) Student BMJ*: student.bmj.com/student/student-bmj.html*
iii) New Scientist*: www.newscientist.com/*

*Example:*

"Having a family member who was diagnosed with lung cancer, I track closely articles on this topic in Nature, New Scientist, and the BMJ; most recently on inhibitors of tyrosine kinase in relation to dealing with mutations caused by the fusion of ALK and EML4 and the encouraging 50-60% response rate. Being involved in this level of scientific discovery, whether the research, testing, or delivery of breakthrough treatments, is a major part of this degree's attraction."

**(b) Dentistry**

i) The Dentist: *http://www.the-dentist.co.uk/subscribe*
ii) Launch Pad (student magazine published by BDA)*: http:// www.bda.org/students/*

*Example:*

"Unable to subscribe to The Dentist magazine myself, I asked my dentist if I could go in each month and copy articles I thought most interesting or that she considered useful to a potential dental student. She agreed and for the last 14 months I have slowly been getting to grips with the technical language involved in dental diseases, procedures, equipment, and practice issues."

**(c) Veterinary Medicine**

i) Scientific American: *www.scientificamerican.com/*
ii) EcoHealth Journal Archive: *https://ecohealth.net/archive.php*
iii) EcoHealth Student (run by two trained vets now focusing on Zoology and Microbiology): *http:// ecohealthstudentsection.weebly.com/* - (plus their Facebook group: *https://www.facebook.com/groups/116366621738000/*)

*Example:*

"A blog post in Scientific American on the serious threat to public health posed by the wild bird trade inspired me to read Wolfe's "The

Viral Storm" to discover more about the spread of viruses from animals to humans. I find this broader application of veterinary science fascinating and have prepared a talk on it for the school's Science Society."

## (d) Nursing

i) Care & Nursing Magazine: *www.careandnursing-magazine.co.uk/*
ii) Nursing Times: *www.nursingtimes.net/*

*Example:*

"The emotional drain on care staff working in palliative care and the measures they must take to protect themselves, which I read about in a recent article in Care & Nursing Magazine, gave me a much better understanding of what this degree will lead to. I appreciate that the degree structure is 50% practical in care-based environments and I will get to learn first-hand, rather than merely theoretically, how to deal with issues such as these."

## 8. Trips / Visits

### (a) Medicine, Dentistry, and Veterinary Medicine

i) Hunterian Collection at the Hunterian Museum: *http://www.rcseng.ac.uk/museums/hunterian/history/collections.html#the-hunterian-collection*
ii) Wellcome Museum of Anatomy and Pathology: *www.rcseng.ac.uk/museums/wellcome/about-the-wellcome-museum-of-anatomy-and-pathology*
iii) The Wellcome Collection: *http://www.wellcomecollection.org/*

The material in the two museums was originally the private collection of John Hunter in the eighteenth century, but was subsequently bought, housed, and separated into various museums by the Royal College of Surgeons and (later) the Wellcome Trust.

Hunter's collection of around 15,000 specimens and preparations formed the nucleus of a still world-renowned museum of comparative anatomy, pathology, osteology, and natural history. The reduced collection today in the Hunterian Collection includes many of Hunter's most famous specimens used for his own medical research into circulation and bone growth.

The Wellcome Musuem is predominantly a teaching and study centre. It contains displays of human bone and tissue prepared to demonstrate a particular aspect of anatomy or pathology. Unusually for a museum, many of the specimens can be handled and examined, and significant degree of support material is provided.

The Wellcome Collection, which is part of the Wellcome Trust, is a free visitor centre, housing exhibitions on the connections between medicine, life, and art.

*Example:*

"A video showing the birth of the first test tube baby at a Wellcome Collection exhibition tied in with the human reproduction component of Biology A-level and was the stimulus for my EPQ subject matter on the long-term consequences of the increasing use of fertility treatment."

iv) The Royal College of Anaesthetists Sixth Form Open Day:
Manchester: *http://www.rcoa.ac.uk/education-and-events/sixth-form-open-day-1*
London: *http://www.rcoa.ac.uk/education-and-events/sixth-form-open-day*

The College runs two Sixth Form Open Days, one in Manchester in December and one in London in February. As well as a lecture, attendees have an opportunity to view and interact with a selection of the technology used by anaesthetists. The lecture is aimed at students who have made their choice of A-level subjects and are considering a career in medicine, but all students who are interested in attending are welcome.

*Example:*

"Applying for the Royal College of Anaesthetists Sixth Form Open Day was a choice I made to understand more about the way in which a medical MDT works together."

v) Odontological Collection in the Hunterian Museum: *www.rcseng.ac.uk/museums/hunterian/history/collections.html#the-odontological-collection*

This separate collection in the museum contains an extensive collection of skulls, jaws, and teeth from humans and hundreds of species of animals, which show normal dental anatomy and a wide range of dental pathologies. For more information, see the Medicine entry above.

*Example:*

"The interplay between dentistry and medicine is exciting, for example the role dentists play in identifying early mouth cancers. Learning about research into dental stigmata of congenital syphilis at the Odontological Collection at the Hunterian Museum further underlined how dentists can help us understand more about a whole range of diseases and I look forward to understanding this in greater depth at degree level."

vi) Body Worlds: *www.bodyworlds.com/en/exhibitions/current_exhibitions.html*

Gunter von Hagens' exhibition of full and dissected bodies, which have undergone "plastination" to preserve them, has become a world-wide phenomenon. For prospective dentistry and medical students, exhibits usefully show detailed human anatomy and the impact of the environment and certain behaviours on the human body.

vii) Pitt-Rivers Museum (Oxford University): www.prm.ox.ac.uk/

This internationally-renowned museum displays archaeological and ethnographic objects from all parts of the world.

*Example:*

"I am scientifically curious and independently visit exhibitions and museums to build my knowledge of scientific history. Two diverse examples are the Bodyworks exhibition, with its detailed examination of the layers that make up human physiology, and the Pitt-Rivers in Oxford, where shrunken heads from Borneo caught my attention. I believe this breadth of interest will serve me well in Dentistry's ongoing learning."

### (b) Nursing

Local schools and nurseries with a specialist focus, such as:

i) Montessori: *www.montessorieducationuk.org*
ii) Steiner Waldorf Schools: www.steinerwaldorf.org

iii) Kumon: *www.kumon.co.uk*
iv) Helen Doron: *www.helendoron.com*

Proactively arranging a visit to a class or institution run by one of these organisations shows your motivation and interest in understanding innovative methods for interacting and helping children - both of which will strengthen your Personal Statement.

*Example:*

"I have independently arranged visits to alternative child education organisations, including a Montessori nursery, a Steiner School, a Kumon class, and a Helen Doron franchise. I have gained a good understanding of different teaching methods and how to effectively engage and establish rapport with young people, vital for this Paediatric Nursing course."

## 9. In-School Activities

Joining or starting a society related to your chosen subject is one of the initiatives I recommend most during Personal Statement workshops and Sixth Form Route-Mapping sessions. This shows all the usual competencies (teamwork, independent research, time management) and can easily give you three lines of content for your Personal Statement. Whether the society organises meetings weekly, fortnightly, or each term, what matters is the wide range of activities that can be talked about in your statement.

Suggested activities for your school society (to name just a few of the options):

i) Individual members research a topic of special interest and give a 15-minute presentation to their peers.
ii) As a group, the society watches a chosen TED talk or other lecture, and then discusses it.
iii) Prominent / successful local people involved in the subject area are invited in to speak.
iv) As a group, the society enters competitions.
v) The society publishes a blog or, once a term, a short newspaper.
vi) The group reads a book or article before the meeting and discusses their thoughts.

### (a) Medicine, Dentistry, and Veterinary Medicine

i) Dissection Society

*Example:*

"Learning the emotional and communication skills to deal with the wide range of human scenarios a vet faces will be stimulating. Founding and running the school Dissection Society and organising sponsorship for my charity runs have provided me with some experience of this. I have learnt to prepare younger students for the shock of actually cutting open a rat or frog, something they think they can handle but often cannot. I have created a process whereby I speak to them individually prior to the dissection, clearly explain what is happening at each stage, and make it easy for them to leave without embarrassment if needed."

ii) Current Ethics Society

*Example:*

"As a doctor would you administer or supervise the death penalty by injection? Under what circumstances would you breach confidentiality? How would you allocate a limited budget amongst possible patient treatment groups? These are three of the topic discussed at the school society I founded. The latter included considering the "Four Box Model" and QALY (quality-adjusted life years). Many students were initially shocked by the fact that it was necessary to make such calculations about people's lives, but at the end of the discussion felt better able to make an informed choice on university and career direction."

iii) Medical Society

*Example:*

"I am the only member of my Sixth Form applying for Dentistry, so I joined the Medical Society rather than establishing anything separate. The two presentations I have given to date covered the physiology of heart disease resulting from cavities in the teeth, and the dentist's role in identifying diseases which can present in the mouth such as cancer, both of which were well received."

iv) Zoology Society

*Example:*

"Effective care of animals requires an understanding of why they behave as they do - part of which involves looking at animals in the wild. To learn more about this, I researched and presented a talk on the behaviour of wild dogs in the Middle East (which I had observed when on a walking holiday with my parents in Oman) for the school's Zoology Society."

## (b) Nursing

i) Health & Social Care Society

*Example:*

"Starting the Health & Social Care Society at my college was daunting. I needed to get the agreement of several senior staff members and to liaise with them regarding room use, time-tabling, and security clearance (CRB) of speakers. Seeing I was serious about wanting to add a new student-driven initiative, they agreed. The most popular talk has been by a midwife on neonatal care."

## 10. Debate Chamber

Attending a Debate Chamber course (£185 for two days) will widen and deepen your understanding of your subject area. It is particularly useful if your university application is likely to involve an interview. The experience will provide you with at least two or three lines of content for your statement, and is often a springboard for additional further reading and more Personal Statement content.

### (a) Medicine

*www.debatechamber.com/summerschools/medicine-summer-school/*

*Example:*

"The ideas I considered at the Debate Chamber Medicine Summer School on obstetrics and paediatrics emphasised how a child's experience at birth and in the first few days of life can have a serious long-term impact on their physical and mental health. How attitudes have changed over the last few decades was particularly fascinating and inspired me to read Donald Winnicot's (now old-fashioned) advice books for mothers. Establishing best practice, constantly improving the quality of care, and in doing so improving the lives of many, is one of the main reasons I want to study this course."

### (b) Dentistry

*www.debatechamber.com/summerschools/dentistry-summer-school/*

*Example:*

"Analysing case studies at the Debate Chamber Dentistry Summer School introduced me to the pathologies dentists deal with on a regular basis and further emphasises the importance of good communication skills,
which I believe I have, in ensuring a positive outcome for the patient."

## 15. Shadowing Programmes and Summer Schools

### (a) Medicine

i) Shadowing at Cambridge University: *http://www.applytocambridge.com/shadowing/*
ii) UNIQ, Oxford University's Summer School for State School Students: *http://www.uniq.ox.ac.uk/*

As with taster days, summer schools, and open days, getting on the Cambridge Shadowing Scheme shows commitment to finding out about university life. As you can imagine, it is highly competitive but Cambridge University is genuinely looking for high-potential candidates from a wide variety of backgrounds. The scheme involves a two-day stay in Cambridge, spending time with a current undergraduate who is studying the subject you are interested in. The whole trip is funded by the university, including accommodation, food, and travel costs (in most cases).

Attending a summer school (usually a week) gives you an insight into university life, an understanding of the type of work that higher level study entails, and concrete ideas on what admissions tutors are looking for when you apply. Run by Oxford University, UNIQ is one of the most competitive summer schools out there. To apply, you will need to submit a mini Personal Statement about your motivation. All of the hints and tips for your UCAS Personal Statement apply equally when writing this. For one-on-one support with writing this, please contact me via my website (www.gwynday.com).

*Example:*

"Being accepted on the University of Cambridge shadowing scheme has confirmed that a challenging course at a leading university is right for me. Sitting in on lectures and lab sessions gave me a real understanding of the difference in standard between A-level and degree-level study. I left very motivated to find out more about my subject, and confident that the independent study and dedication required at university play to my strengths."

*Or:*

"As the first person in my family to attend university, I was apprehensive before attending the week-long Oxford University UNIQ summer school. During my time there, I was fascinated by the breadth of subject matter on offer in Medicine (including my particular area of interest - oncology) and excited by the variety of student life. I am now certain that this style of focused course is best for me."

**(b) Veterinary Medicine**

i) Shadowing at Cambridge University (see Medicine above): *http://www.applytocambridge.com/shadowing/*
ii) Shadowing Day at Royal Veterinary College (University of London): *www.rvc.ac.uk/widening-participation/StudentShadowing.cfm*

In a bid to widen access, the Royal Veterinary College offers shadowing placements for students in Year 12 and 13 from state schools whose families have no history of going to university. Students spend a day shadowing a current undergraduate, attending the student's classes and lectures, taking part in practical work and talking to them about their course and university experiences.

*Example:*

"Without a network of people to ask - my family has no history of university study and I am the first person in my school to apply for this course - I independently researched and applied for the Royal Veterinary College's student shadowing placement. Attending two lectures and a dissection class with a second-year undergraduate, and discussing her experiences over lunch, reassured me that I would thrive in this pressured, academic environment."

## OTHER RELEVANT ACTIVITIES RELEVANT FOR ALL DISCIPLINES

### 16. University Open Days and Taster Days

The end of the summer term is the best time to attend these, not the autumn when you are under pressure from the increased workload of A2 (or equivalent). When talking about your time at open days in your Personal Statement, be sure to say you went with a mission to understand what the course would be like and to detail how the trip confirmed or reinforced your conviction to apply to university.

Subject-specific university experience days are fantastic proof that you are serious about choosing the right course for you. Why? Places on these days disappear very quickly and the fact that you applied early enough to get a place shows forethought, research skills, and time management.

## 17. EPQ (Extended Project Qualification)

*http://www.aqa.org.uk/programmes/aqa-baccalaureate/extended-project/the-aqa-epq*

If your school offered this opportunity, I hope you decided to take it. This can easily be worth six lines or even a full paragraph of a Personal Statement. Given that the qualification involves considerable reading and the determination to complete a 4,000 word essay to university standard in your own time, it clearly indicates the calibre of person you are. What is important about the EPQ is that you can choose any topic and this allows you to explore, compare, and contrast ideas on an area of science, relevant to your subject, which really interests you, and to form your own opinion. When it comes to your Personal Statement, you should mention the relevant EPQ-related books, lectures, and even interviews you may have arranged.

## 18. Prizes

Prizes - whether at school, regional, national, or international level - show that you are prepared to compete. Universities want students to be driving for a First in their degree studies and will be impressed that you are willing to be tested voluntarily and to put yourself under pressure.

## 19. Maths / Biology / Physics / Chemistry Olympiads

If you get a medal or award, this is a great way of showing you have the requisite skills in the subjects required for your chosen degree. If you do not do well, then no need to mention it.

British Maths Olympiad: *http://www.ukmt.org.uk/individual-competitions/british-mathematical-olympiad/*
British Physics Olympiad: *http://www.physics.ox.ac.uk/olympiad/index.html*
British Chemistry Olympiad: *http://www.rsc.org/Education/events-and-competitions/Olympiad/About.asp*
British Biology Olympiad: *http://ukbiologycompetitions.org/british-biology-olympiad/*
UK Maths Challenge: *http://www.ukmt.org.uk/individual-competitions/*

## 20. Peer Subject Coach / Private Tutor

Universities know that the best way to understand a subject is to teach it. If you can break a topic or concept down and successfully explain it to others, then you will surely understand it yourself. Knowing how to do that will make it easier for you to grasp new concepts at university. For prospective dentists and from an entrepreneurial perspective, running your own tutoring business gives you a superb understanding of the business theory you will need when running a practice of your own.

## 21. Subject Ambassador

This is another area I strongly encourage in the schools I visit. If this does not exist in your school or Sixth Form College, get it set up. Being a Subject Ambassador means giving talks to both parents and students (individually and together) to promote your subject and convince them of the benefits of studying it at GCSE or A-level (or its equivalent). Universities will definitely appreciate that you enjoy the subject so much that you are prepared to promote it. The soft skills you develop doing so are an added bonus.

## 22. Listening to Radio 4

Health-specific programmes, such as "Inside Health", "The Why Factor", and "All in the Mind", provide very different viewpoints on current and historical matters linked to your subject. More general programmes, such as "In Our Time" and "Farming Today" frequently cover relevant hot topics for Veterinary Medicine applicants. Few Sixth Formers listen to these and mentioning them will make you stand out.

i) Inside Health: *http://www.bbc.co.uk/programmes/b019dl1b*
ii) The Why Factor: *http://www.bbc.co.uk/programmes/p01vzjrz*
iii) All in the Mind: *http://www.bbc.co.uk/programmes/b04795vc*
iv) In Our Time: *http://www.bbc.co.uk/programmes/p00545f8*
v) Farming Today: *http://www.bbc.co.uk/programmes/b006qj8q*

## Chapter 7

# Personal Statement Paragraph 4: NON SUBJECT-SPECIFIC ACTIVITIES

In paragraph 4 you will write about your non subject-related activities. This may sound easy compared to other sections in the statement, but actually requires just as much careful thought.

Students often write a long shopping list of activities to demonstrate how busy and active they are. Far more interesting to admissions tutors, however, is to see that you have done one or two activities for an extended period of time, and taken them to a high level of achievement. Again, the "what" is not that important, but the "how" of having shown commitment and improvement over several years is.

You may have your own examples already. If you do not, choose no more than two or three from the list below which are relevant to you. For each activity, work out the skills you developed and how these skills will help you at university and/or in your chosen course. This information is what you need to write down.

Given the weight you will give in your statement to work experience and voluntary work, you may find that that you have very little space, if any at all, to devote to non subject-specific activities. There is nothing wrong with this. As you will see from Example Statement 1 in Chapter 10, your statement does not need a whole list of hobbies to make it compelling.

****PLAGIARISM ALERT****

### 1. Sport

*Example:*

"As a break from my studies I play cricket and would like to play for the university team. Playing for the school and the county has instilled self-discipline. I know that if I do not turn up to practice or to a match because I am tired or have homework, I will be letting others down, and, consequently, I have learnt to organise my studies effectively."

*Or:*

"My serious hobby outside of school is karate. In five years, I have reached Brown Belt, and will be taking the Black Belt this summer. It gives me a feeling of concentration and control, which I think will help me in stressful situations in my future career."

### 2. Music

*Example:*

"Achieving Grade 8 on the violin represents five years' commitment and progress. Preparing for and playing in concerts has helped my attention to detail and focus, as I need to be constantly aware of what is happening and adapt to unexpected changes. Performing solos (the largest audience was 300) has built confidence in my ability to achieve what I set out to do."

*Or:*

"Performing a violin solo in front of 300 people was the culmination of reaching Grade 8 and five years of hard work. I fully commit to whatever I start, and this same sense of achievement is what I expect when I graduate."

### 3. Drama

*Example:*

"My main interest away from academics is acting. I have taken multiple LAMDA qualifications over the past five years. Acting lead roles in front of hundreds of people and public speaking in debates has given me confidence in my communication skills, and so much more. Preparing for roles, whether in school or my drama school, has taught me to how better to relate to other people, trying to understand what motivates them, why they behave as they do, and how they will react to me. This has given me a strong sense of empathy, which I think will transfer well to the clinical side of Medicine."

*Or:*

"Playing Othello in a youth amateur dramatics society in front of 150 people showed me that I had conquered my fears of speaking in public. Three years ago I heard through family friends that most degrees require project work and formal presentations; I hated public speaking but was determined to be the first in my family to attend university. I volunteered for the school play and, from there, took LAMDA exams and joined other theatre projects. I am at the point where I enjoy acting but, more importantly, the experience has taught me that if I rise to the challenge I can successfully achieve my goals."

## 4. Duke of Edinburgh's Award

*Example:*

"Getting my Silver Duke of Edinburgh's Award, and particularly completing the expedition, was a significant achievement for me, both because I am from an inner city school and rarely spend time in the countryside and because I suffer from asthma. My team helped me a lot, and I learned the value of supporting others to achieve their best. From research I have seen that this course involves project work, often with diverse groups, and I think the DofE experience will greatly help with this."

*Or:*

“Aside from academics, my greatest achievement at school has been completing all three Duke of Edinburgh's Awards. The Expedition for my Gold Award was in the Black Mountains in Wales. The weather turned against us badly and one of the team had asthma attacks. As a learning experience of decision-making under pressure and the importance of getting group consensus, I think it will be a major help in my future.”

## 5. Part-time job

*Example:*

“For the last two years I have worked part-time as a waitress in my local pub and will continue full-time over my AS and A2 summer holidays. I am saving what I earn because I want to enjoy myself at university, try new activities, and graduate with as little debt as possible. Being responsible for ten tables with sometimes up to 40 customers means good organisation, diplomacy when things go wrong, and willpower to keep going.”

*Or:*

“Dealing with sometimes angry customers, taking responsibility for cashing up hundreds or thousands of pounds, and training new staff have been aspects of my waitressing job for the last two years. I took the job as I want to be as financially independent as possible and graduate from university with lower debt than most. Considered by my employers as highly efficient and reliable, I have been offered full-time work in the pub whenever I want, an offer which I will take up this (AS) summer and next."

## 6. Self-employment

*Example:*

"A year ago I started my own business buying and selling items I think teenagers want - from iPhone covers to t-shirts. I negotiate with suppliers I find online and then market the products through my social media network. Juggling my time and dealing with the many small problems which occur have shown me how important attention to detail and thinking ahead are in business."

*Or:*

"Running my own part-time business repairing screens on iPhones and iPads for the last two years has required delicate practical skills, as well as learning how to deal with people. On work experience placements, I observed that dentists must adapt their manner to suit the patient, especially when treating children or the elderly. With customers in my own business - often older people worried about expense - I think I have developed the foundations for a clear and reassuring communication style so essential to this profession."

## 7. CCF (Combined Cadet Forces)

*Example:*

"While not considering a career in the Armed Forces, I joined the CCF for the personal development opportunities it offers. Now leading a platoon, I understand a lot more about what it takes to organise others and how that is only possible if I am efficient and detail-oriented myself."

*Or:*

"I feel I am ready for the demands of university and much of that is due to my involvement in the CCF. The self-discipline required, whether looking after equipment or during drills and exercises, has instilled in me a strong work ethic. I have learnt to organise my time efficiently and get tasks done before, rather than on, the deadline. Since becoming Platoon Leader I have greatly improved my communication, leadership, and decision-making skills, most notably when dealing with and motivating younger cadets. Knowing how to achieve my goals will help me meet the challenge of this degree."

## 8. Community Involvement

*Example:*

"I have been involved with the Scouting movement for ten years. The responsibilities I have taken on have involved motivating, leading, and supporting others. Experiences such as taking groups of cubs from urban areas on summer country camps - both exciting and, at times, unnerving - have developed my decision-making, public-speaking, and lateral-thinking skills, all of which will be useful on this course."

*Or:*

"As a member of the Hindu faith, I take great pleasure in giving back to a community which gives me so much. The two activities I divide my attention between are working with the elderly infirm and helping mentally handicapped children. In both cases I have learnt patience, especially in finding different ways of communicating. Most importantly, I know how wrong it is to prejudge people and how there is something to learn from everyone - an attitude which I will apply in university life."

## 9. Political Involvement

*Example:*

"For the last year I have been involved with the Muslim Youth Council of Great Britain. I attend meetings which discuss issues both within the Muslim community and concerning links with the wider world. I am especially proud of a presentation I gave on how to encourage more Muslims to cycle to work and college rather than taking public transport or driving. At university I want to help promote diversity, and would love to become an Ambassador reaching out to prospective applicants."

*Or:*

"I am and will continue to be politically active. I believe in diversity, but since the end of Aim Higher funding and the introduction of higher university fees, I have seen a drop in the number of young Muslims in my community applying to university. Through involvement in the Muslim Youth Council of Great Britain, I have spoken at several community events in my borough to raise aspiration and promote further education."

## 10. Charity Work / Volunteering

*Example:*

"I started volunteering at my local Cancer Research shop after several relatives were diagnosed with this illness. I am impressed by the dedication that goes into the research for a cure and the care given by organisations to people with this condition. I only work four hours a week but feel all contributions make a difference. After speaking to customers with cancer, I trained for and completed a half marathon, raising £300 which I donated to my local shop."

*Or:*

"As a hobby I enjoy running and have completed multiple 5k and 10k races and two half marathons. Though I run predominantly for fun and exercise, to date I have raised over £4,000 for the RSPCA and WWF. I volunteer weekly at the local RSPCA shelter, where I have learnt how easily animal behaviour patterns can be modified by mistreatment or caring treatment."

## 11. Other Hobbies

*Example:*

"In my spare time I play traditional Indian musical instruments, such as the sita. I give performances locally, both individually and as part of a group. While being open and international in outlook (I want to be involved in the Erasmus Programme at university), I believe it is important to have a connection with my culture's traditions. Since starting five years ago, I have now achieved proficiency and continue to practise every day."

*Or:*

"I build rockets as my hobby. I enjoy the research and problem-solving involved in getting the rocket to go higher or further each time without increasing the size, and am part of an online community which exchanges ideas and tips. Going to rocket fairs I have made friends nationally and internationally. Thinking about how to continuously improve and refine my work is a skill which will transfer well to university."

### 12. Travel

*Example:*

"Travelling internationally with my family, school, and independently has opened my eyes to how lucky we are in the UK. While citizens do have real problems, they are minor when compared to what faces so many others globally. My family originally comes from Nigeria. Trips there and to neighbouring countries have motivated me to push myself academically and use the resources available to me. I know there are millions of children who would love to have access to the education I have, but are prevented by circumstance."

*Or:*

"Coming to Britain three years ago from Kazakhstan has involved overcoming major language and cultural obstacles. I think the perspective I have gained from knowing two completely different worlds has made me more flexible and understanding in my approach to others."

### 13. Prefect / School Positions

*Example:*

"Being appointed a Prefect has given me my first taste of organising, managing, and motivating others. One of my duties is speaking in assembly and at some parent events. This has built my sense of responsibility and made me confident about speaking in front of others."

*Or:*

"I am proud of my involvement in the school's Charity Committee, where I am the Treasurer and report directly to the School Bursar. Part of our work involves organising approximately six events each year. Last year we donated over £5,000 to two schools in Uganda, with whom we are twinned. As Treasurer, I keep the accounts and arrange the distribution of funds for equipment required at events. One of my biggest jobs is chasing people for paperwork and accurate numbers."

## 14. Head Boy / Head Girl

*Example:*

"Being elected Head Girl by my peers and the Senior Leadership Team required a review of my achievements and contributions, and several public speeches to explain to the school body what I thought I could bring to the role. I direct a team of ten prefects and we are included in consultations regarding changes which impact Years 12 and 13. I have given several speeches to parents of existing and potential students. This combination of leadership, teamwork, and getting things done should help me successfully contribute to university life."

*Or:*

"I believe I was elected as Head Boy for two main reasons. Firstly, I get on with a wide range of students, including rugby team mates, choir friends, and Medicine Society peers. Secondly, I get things done and am not afraid to lobby and approach senior staff if the situation requires it: e.g. in Year 11 I initiated links between our school rugby team and an under-performing school in our area."

## Chapter 8

# Personal Statement Paragraph 5: WRAPPING UP

The final paragraph of your Personal Statement is the easiest. In it you need to cover at least two of the four suggested points below. Aim for between two and three lines in length - short and sweet is definitely best.

You can:

1. Summarise what you have already said to demonstrate you are a good fit for the course.

2. Refer to some of the specific skills that your first choice universities have said you will gain or develop during the degree.

3. Mention your understanding of the specifics of career path options outlined on university websites.

4. Talk about broader professional / academic opportunities you will hope to take advantage of during course.

****PLAGIARISM ALERT****

## Medicine

*Example (demonstrating points 1 and 2):*

"Based on my work experience at hospitals and volunteering, further academic research from books and articles in the Junior BMJ and New Scientist, and what I learnt attending during MedSim at Nottingham University and the Debate Chamber Advanced Medicine course, I am dedicated to this subject and profession and look forward to the challenges and rewards ahead."

*Or (demonstrating points 1 and 2):*

"I am highly motivated by the problem-based-learning structure your Medical School provides, and hope that, with my deep-rooted academic interest, strong personal skills, and independent motivation, you see my profile as suitable for this course."

## Dentistry

*Example (demonstrating points 1 and 3):*

"I am confident that I have the academic ability and drive required to successfully pursue a dentistry career and hope that my commitment and focus in preparing this application over an extended period of time prove I deserve a place on your course."

## Veterinary Science

*Example (demonstrating points 1, 2 and 4):*

"Attending university taster days and Vetsim have assured me that I can rise to the academic demands of the course, and my work experiences have proved that I will cope with the physical, mental, and emotional aspects involved. I have already looked at the opportunities available via student BVA membership and will take full advantage if offered a place."

## Nursing

*Example (demonstrating points 1 and 3):*

"I am a caring and compassionate person, who can get things done. I am highly motivated to do well on your course and to use the opportunities it will give me to gain skills, with a particular focus on child and community nursing."

## Chapter 9

# REFINING YOUR PERSONAL STATEMENT TO MAKE IT UNIQUE

By this point you will have the basic content of your Personal Statement mapped out. Now you must refine it and make it more personal. This chapter will help you.

The steps below aim not to add in further information on books you have read or accolades you have collected; instead, they show you how to improve the language and tweak the structure to leverage the work you have already done, and ultimately make your Personal Statement unique to you.

Follow each step carefully, and allow yourself time to experiment with structure and various turns of phrase.

****PLAGIARISM ALERT****

**Step 1: Take your almost finished draft and split it into sections. Label each section to establish exactly what it adds to your statement and what it proves about you as an applicant to admissions tutors. See the example statement and the labels in *italics* below.**

*Example Draft Personal Statement*

Paragraph 1 / Reason for choosing course

*[Specific trigger with detailed academic interest / aptitude]*
It has been the more detailed study of Chemistry at A-level and beyond which has helped my decision to study Medicine at university. Learning about the processes and mechanisms of organic chemistry has underlined how it should be possible to treat the vast majority of illnesses and diseases.

Paragraph 2 / Evidence of interest in and aptitude for subject, using further reading

*[Evidence 1: Further reading and how it has strengthened commitment to this course]*
My interest has been reinforced by reading books such as "Why Chemical Reactions Happen" and "Power, Sex, Suicide", making me want to both learn more and apply my knowledge in a clinical setting.

*[Evidence 2: How Biology has stimulated specific medical interest, studied in-depth in relevant EPQ]*
Studying Biology in parallel has given me a broader perspective, part of which involved doing the obligatory AS Biology extended coursework and an EPQ. The latter was most interesting for me because I could choose the exact parameters of the essay, "An investigation into the potential health consequences of the Paleo Diet".

*[Evidence 2: Independent research for EPQ showing suitability for independent study]*
Self-directing my EPQ research, I referenced six scientific papers, two longitudinal studies, and numerous books and articles. I even independently arranged international phone interviews. My conclusion was that this diet has been maligned far more than the specific health results merit. I look forward to doing similar, but more demanding, research-led work at university.

*[Evidence 3: EPQ stimulated more further reading and helped form own opinion on public health]*
The EPQ sparked my interest in the correlation between legislating against tobacco and, in the future, against sugar. I follow this debate closely in the scientific and broadsheet press. As in the 1960s, medical opinion on the obesity epidemic in Britain is becoming increasingly politicised. As Boswell writes in "The Shape We're In", working on the frontline, doctors across many disciplines - e.g. psychology, cardiology, bariatric surgery - are urging government to see obesity as more than a matter of individual responsibility and bring out legislation that helps people stop consuming such large quantities of sugar.

<u>Paragraph 3 / Further evidence of interest and aptitude, using subject-specific extracurricular activities</u>

*[Evidence 1: Work experience and how this changed attitude to aspect of medicine]*
Observing a Consultant in the ENT Department at a major teaching hospital made me realise the serious implications of a procedure

often considered a joke. There were several patients who wanted to have rhinoplasty. Having spoken to patients and the Consultant, I see that rhinoplasty can definitely be a necessary medical procedure for both physical and mental reasons. What seemed absurd, having to decide if the patient is really suffering or just wants cosmetic surgery at NHS expense, is now something I see as a serious budgetary and ethical decision.

*[Evidence 2: Work experience and ethical debate it prompted student to think about]*
A two-week placement in a local Neonatal Unit introduced me to the incredibly skilled application of medicine on such tiny bodies, while highlighting the serious ethical debate which comes with the costly staff-to-patient ratio and the complex machinery required.

*[Evidence 3: Competitions and how they prove suitability for course]*
I have competed in several science competitions, including the team-based "Top of the Bench", the Royal Society of Chemistry Bill Bryson Prize, and the Biology Olympiad (achieving a gold medal both years). Taking part in these competitions allows me to think more creatively and apply my knowledge independently, without being helped or directed by a teacher - a beneficial experience for university study.

Paragraph 4 / Other extracurricular, unrelated to subject but evidencing useful qualities

*[Evidence 1: Drama and how this has developed skills required in this challenging degree/career.]*
My main interest away from academics is acting. I have taken multiple LAMDA qualifications over the past five years. Acting lead roles and public speaking in debates has given me confidence in my communication skills, and much more.

*[Evidence 2: Other relevant skills drama has developed - e.g. empathy]*
Preparing for roles has taught me to how to relate to other people, trying to understand what motivates them, why they behave as they do, and how they will react to me. This has given me a strong sense of empathy, which I think will transfer well to the clinical side of Medicine.

*[Evidence 3: commitment to drama and awareness of how rigorous course is]*
Though I am fully aware of the academic demands of Medicine as a degree and this will always come first, my goal is to continue acting at university when possible.

Paragraph 5 / Wrap up

*[Reference to specific type of course, and reiteration of academic interest and motivation]*

I am highly motivated by the problem-based-learning structure your Medical School provides, and hope that, with my deep-rooted academic interest, strong personal skills, and independent motivation, you see my profile as suitable for this course.

**Step 2: Move around the sections to give your Personal Statement the shape you want.**

*Reworked Example 1:*

It has been the more detailed study of Chemistry at A-level and beyond which has helped my decision to study Medicine at university. My interest has been reinforced by reading books such as "Why Chemical Reactions Happen" and "Power, Sex, Suicide", making me want to both learn more and apply my knowledge in a clinical setting.

Learning about the processes and mechanisms of organic chemistry has underlined how it should be possible to treat the vast majority of illnesses and diseases. Studying Biology in parallel has given me a broader perspective, part of which involved doing the obligatory AS Biology extended coursework and an EPQ. The latter was most interesting for me because I could choose the exact parameters of the essay, "An investigation into the potential health consequences of the Paleo Diet".

The EPQ sparked my interest in the correlation between legislating against tobacco and, in the future, against sugar. I follow this debate closely in the scientific and broadsheet press. As in the 1960s, medical opinion on the obesity epidemic in Britain is becoming increasingly politicised. As Boswell writes in "The Shape We're In", working on the frontline, doctors across many disciplines - e.g. psychology, cardiology, bariatric surgery - are urging government to see obesity as more than a matter of individual responsibility and bring out legislation that helps people stop consuming such large quantities of sugar.

Self-directing my EPQ research, I referenced six scientific papers, two longitudinal studies, and numerous books and articles. I even independently arranged international phone interviews. My conclusion was that this diet has been maligned far more than the specific health results merit. I look forward to doing similar, but more demanding, research-led work at university.

I have competed in several science competitions, including the team-based "Top of the Bench", the Royal Society of Chemistry Bill Bryson Prize, and the Biology Olympiad (achieving a gold medal both years). Taking part in these competitions allows me to think more creatively and apply my knowledge independently, without being helped or directed by a teacher - a beneficial experience for university study.

A two-week placement in a local Neonatal Unit introduced me to the incredibly skilled application of medicine on such tiny bodies, while highlighting the serious ethical debate which comes with the costly staff-to-patient ratio and the complex machinery required. Observing a Consultant in the ENT Department at a major teaching hospital made me realise the serious implications of a procedure often considered a joke. There were several patients who wanted to have rhinoplasty. Having spoken to patients and the Consultant, I see that rhinoplasty can definitely be a necessary medical procedure for both physical and mental reasons. What seemed absurd, having to decide if the patient is really suffering or just wants cosmetic surgery at NHS expense, is now something I see as a serious budgetary and ethical decision.

My main interest away from academics is acting. I have taken multiple LAMDA qualifications over the past five years. Though I am fully aware of the academic demands of Medicine as a degree and this will always come first, my goal is to continue acting at university when possible. Acting lead roles and public speaking in debates has given me confidence in my communication skills, and much more. Preparing for roles has taught me to how to relate to other people, trying to understand what motivates them, why they behave as they do, and how they will react to me. This has given me a strong sense of empathy, which I think will transfer well to the clinical side of Medicine.

I am highly motivated by the problem-based-learning structure your Medical School provides, and hope that, with my deep-rooted academic interest, strong personal skills, and independent motivation, you see my profile as suitable for this course.

*Reworked Example 2:*

Learning about the processes and mechanisms of organic chemistry has underlined how it should be possible to treat the vast majority of illnesses and diseases. It has been the more detailed study of Chemistry at A-level and beyond which has helped my decision to study Medicine at university. My interest has been reinforced by reading books such as "Why Chemical Reactions Happen" and "Power, Sex, Suicide", making me want to both learn more and apply my knowledge in a clinical setting.

A two-week placement in a local Neonatal Unit introduced me to the incredibly skilled application of medicine on such tiny bodies, while highlighting the serious ethical debate which comes with the costly staff-to-patient ratio and the complex machinery required. Observing a Consultant in the ENT Department at a major teaching hospital made me realise the serious implications of a procedure often considered a joke. There were several patients who wanted to have rhinoplasty. Having spoken to patients and the Consultant, I see that rhinoplasty can definitely be a necessary medical procedure for both physical and mental reasons. What seemed absurd, having to decide if the patient is really suffering or just wants cosmetic surgery at NHS expense, is now something I see as a serious budgetary and ethical decision.

Studying Biology in parallel has given me a broader perspective, part of which involved doing the obligatory AS Biology extended coursework and an EPQ. The latter was most interesting for me because I could choose the exact parameters of the essay, "An investigation into the potential health consequences of the Paleo Diet". Self-directing my EPQ research, I referenced six scientific papers, two longitudinal studies, and numerous books and articles. I even independently arranged international phone interviews. My conclusion was that this diet has been maligned far more than the specific health results merit. The EPQ sparked my interest in the correlation between legislating against tobacco and, in the future, against sugar. I follow this debate closely in the scientific and broadsheet press. As in the 1960s, medical opinion on the obesity epidemic in Britain is becoming increasingly politicised. As Boswell writes in "The Shape We're In", working on the frontline, doctors across many disciplines - e.g. psychology, cardiology, bariatric surgery - are urging government to see obesity as more than a matter of individual responsibility and bring out legislation that helps people stop consuming such large quantities of sugar. I look forward to doing similar, but more demanding, research-led work at university.

My main interest away from academics is acting. I have taken multiple LAMDA qualifications over the past five years. Acting lead roles and public speaking in debates has given me confidence in my communication skills, and much more. Preparing for roles has taught me to how to relate to other people, trying to understand what motivates them, why they behave as they do, and how they will react to me. This has given me a strong sense of empathy, which I think will transfer well to the clinical side of Medicine. Though I am fully aware of the academic demands of Medicine as a degree and this will always come first, my goal is to continue acting at university when possible.

I have competed in several science competitions, including the team-based "Top of the Bench", the Royal Society of Chemistry Bill Bryson Prize, and the Biology Olympiad (achieving a gold medal both years). Taking part in these competitions allows me to think more creatively and apply my knowledge independently, without being helped or directed by a teacher - a beneficial experience for university study.

I am highly motivated by the problem-based-learning structure your Medical School provides, and hope, with my deep-rooted academic interest, strong personal skills, and independent motivation, that you see my profile as suitable for this course.

**Step 3: Having found a sequence you like, start changing / replacing words in your statement to make it uniquely yours. The highlighted words in the example statement can be replaced with the suggested options in the table below. Use this process as a guide for how to refine your own statement.**

*(NOTE: Though you will still think of your Personal Statement in terms of "blocks" of content, you will not use paragraph indentations or even new lines on the online UCAS form. As mentioned, this is because the 4000 character limit simply does not leave you enough space to do so.)*

It has been the more detailed study of Chemistry at A-level and beyond which has helped my decision to study Medicine at university. Learning about the processes and mechanisms of organic chemistry has underlined how it should be possible to treat the vast majority of illnesses and diseases.

My interest has been reinforced by reading books such as "Why Chemical Reactions Happen" and "Power, Sex, Suicide", making me want to both learn more and apply my knowledge in a clinical setting. Studying Biology in parallel has given me a broader perspective, part of which involved doing the obligatory AS Biology extended coursework and an EPQ. The latter was most interesting for me because I could choose the exact parameters of the essay, "An investigation into the potential health consequences of the Paleo Diet". Self-directing my EPQ research, I referenced six scientific papers, two longitudinal studies, and numerous books and articles. I even independently arranged international phone interviews. My conclusion was that this diet has been maligned far more than the specific health results merit. I look forward to doing similar, but more demanding, research-led work at university.

The EPQ sparked my interest in the correlation between legislating against tobacco and, in the future, against sugar. I follow this debate closely in the scientific and broadsheet press. As in the 1960s, medical opinion on the obesity epidemic in Britain is becoming increasingly politicised. As Boswell writes in "The Shape We're In", working on the frontline, doctors across many disciplines - e.g. psychology, cardiology, bariatric surgery - are urging government to see obesity as more than a matter of individual responsibility and bring out legislation that helps people stop consuming such large quantities of sugar.

Observing a Consultant in the ENT Department at a major teaching hospital made me realise the serious implications of a procedure often considered a joke. There were several patients who wanted to have rhinoplasty. Having spoken to patients and the Consultant, I see that rhinoplasty can definitely be a necessary medical procedure for both physical and mental reasons. What seemed absurd, having to decide if the patient is really suffering or just wants cosmetic surgery at NHS expense, is now something I see as a serious budgetary and ethical decision. A two-week placement in a local Neonatal Unit introduced me to the incredibly skilled application of medicine on such tiny bodies, while highlighting the serious ethical debate which comes with the costly staff-to-patient ratio and the complex machinery required.

I have competed in several science competitions, including the team-based "Top of the Bench", the Royal Society of Chemistry Bill Bryson Prize, and the Biology Olympiad (achieving a gold medal both years). Taking part in these competitions allows me to think more creatively and apply my knowledge independently, without being helped or directed by a teacher - a beneficial experience for university study.

My main interest away from academics is acting. I have taken multiple LAMDA qualifications over the past five years. Acting lead roles and public speaking in debates has given me confidence in my communication skills, and much more. Preparing for roles has taught me to how to relate to other people, trying to understand what motivates them, why they behave as they do, and how they will react to me. This has given me a strong sense of empathy, which I think will transfer well to the clinical side of Medicine. Though I am fully aware of the academic demands of Medicine as a degree and this will always come first, my goal is to continue acting at university when possible.

I am highly motivated by the problem-based-learning structure your Medical School provides, and hope that, with my deep-rooted academic interest, strong personal skills, and independent motivation, you see my profile as suitable for this course.

**Other phrasing options and sample vocabulary:**

Use the suggested variations below to tweak your Personal Statement and make the language less repetitive and more expressive.

| | |
|---|---|
| detailed | in depth, complex, comprehensive, precise |
| has helped my | has encouraged my, has motivated me, prompted, moved me towards the |
| learning about | studying, understanding, unravelling, unpicking |
| underlined | emphasised, brought me to see, helped me see |
| my interest has been reinforced by X | X has made me more certain that, X gave me even more confidence that |
| in parallel | at the same time, together with this, over the same period |

| broader perspective | wider view, greater understanding, a bigger scientific spectrum |
|---|---|
| choose | determine, decide on, set, dictate |
| self-directing | choosing my own, setting the course for my own, being in control of, being responsible for |
| has been maligned | has been criticised, is discredited, has been dismissed |
| I look forward to | I am motivated by the prospect of, I am excited by the opportunity to |
| sparked my interest | made me think about, prompted me to consider, opened my eyes to |
| is becoming increasingly politicised | takes on an greater political edge, is becoming more politically motivated, is more and more in the political sphere |
| urging | encouraging, asking, campaigning for |
| bring out legislation | legislate, act decisively, change the law |
| observing | shadowing, doing a work placement with, on placement with |
| often considered a joke | not always taken seriously, frequently dismissed, not always fairly appreciated |
| having spoken to | following conversations with, talking to, hearing the perspective of |
| a serious budgetary and ethical decision | with serious budgetary and ethical implications, important in terms of budget and ethics, something which should be seriously considered from financial and ethical standpoints |
| introduced me to | showed me, helped me see, made me aware of, was my first insight into |

| | |
|---|---|
| taking part in | competing in, going in for, being a competitor at, participating in |
| my main interest away from academics | outside of school my focus is, aside from academic work a major priority is, my primary activity beyond school and Medicine is |
| I have taken multiple | I have completed a number of, I have achieved X up to X, I have successfully done |
| has given me confidence in | has helped me improve, has strengthened my, has developed my |
| has taught me | has given me a better sense of, has shown me, is a good insight into |
| given me a strong sense of empathy | made me more empathetic, made me think more about how people feel, given me a developed understanding of other people's feelings |
| will transfer well to | highly transferable to, applies itself well to, will help with |
| academic demands | rigours of, how taxing X is, the intellectual challenges involved |
| deep-rooted academic interest | highly developed academic interest, intellectual commitment, fascination with the subject |
| suitable for this course | the right fit for, a viable candidate for, the highly-qualified candidate you are looking for |

## Chapter 10:

# SEVEN EXAMPLES OF PERSONAL STATEMENTS

By this stage your Personal Statement will be taking shape. Now spend some time comparing it to the examples of strong Personal Statements below and see if you need to make any further changes.

The example statements are divided into the sections detailed in Chapter 2. This is to show you the thought process behind each one. As mentioned, when you submit your own statement via UCAS, it will not be spaced like this because of the character limit.

In the examples, each section is labelled to show you what is being addressed, what that proves about the student, and how much "space" this idea is given. If your statement is well structured, you will be able to break it down in a similar way.

****PLAGIARISM ALERT****

### EXAMPLE 1 - MEDICINE

*(NOTE: This statement includes such a wealth of work experience and subject-specific extracurricular activities that there is no space nor reason to include any non subject-specific activities (Paragraph 4 - e.g. sport, drama). This is fine. The impact of the relevant material is far greater than anything else.)*

Paragraph 1

*[Reason for applying: academic and career goal]*
First-hand experience of care-giving and in-depth scientific study, far beyond the scope of my A-level syllabus, instigated and confirmed my conviction to pursue a career in the medical profession and take Medicine as my first degree.

Paragraph 2

*[Further reading 1: combined with work experience observations and displaying scientific knowledge]*
Encountering the complexity of opportunistic cancers in HIV clinics while observing the Oncology Department's MDT at St James Hospital (Newcastle) showed me how diverse even a specialised area of Medicine can be and the reality of "life-long learning". Discussing cell signalling in more detail with the consultant led me to read Leroi's "Mutants" and subsequently research the most frequently disrupted pathways when cancers are present, such as IGF.

*[Further reading 2: combined with volunteering, personal view on medical approaches, and broader public health issues]*
Alongside advancements in conventional Medicine, I am convinced by the importance of preventative care. A common theme when talking to elderly patients at a local clinic, at which I volunteer, is regret at not being more active when younger. These patients believe (and in my opinion, rightly) that better physical condition in their youth would have prevented, or at least improved, their

mobility issues and chronic conditions, such as high blood pressure and type 2 diabetes. Far greater investment on a national scale, spear-headed by the medical community, will be essential for improving health standards in Britain. Boswell's "The Shape We're In" confirmed my view on the need for greater for legislation in the soft drinks and snack food industries. The role doctors play in making the public health case for this to government is one of my motivations for studying this course.

Paragraph 3

*[Subject-specific activity 1: TED talks linking to motivation to study course]*
From my wider research I am increasingly aware that there are still many unknown influences on physical and mental health. This exploration of new ideas and the bringing together of seemingly disparate elements to enhance quality of life is a fascinating facet of Medicine. To improve my own understanding beyond A-level and my further reading, I watch the latest TED talks; for example, Amy Cuddy's talk on how positive body language triggers chemical changes which actually result in a more positive outlook and confidence has huge consequences, whether for those attending interviews or more importantly for those suffering mild depression.

*[Subject-specific activity 2: MedSoc linked to more further reading]*
A significant aspect of Medicine's appeal is the responsibility involved in being the decision-maker and the required ethical understanding to make difficult choices. I have looked at the 4 Box

Method and feel that, while it is a useful model, it requires a strong philosophical underpinning. Reading Carey's "The Epigenetics Revolution" and Ruse's "The Philosophy of Biology" contributed another level to my understanding of the BMC's ethical guidelines. I have introduced some of these topics to other students through my role as Chair of the school Medical Society. To promote membership to the incoming Year 12, I got permission to run a one-off 'Dissection Lunchtime', which was the best attended MedSoc event ever and has ensured strong attendance this term.

*[Subject-specific activity 3: St John's Ambulance, explaining how this experience deepened interest in course]*
For the last three years, I have been a member of St John's Ambulance. Using the skills taught twice - both while volunteering at my local football stadium - has increased my determination to study Medicine. In the first instance, a man had an epileptic fit, and, in the second, a child fainted (as a result of heat and dehydration). In both cases I responded quickly and provided first aid until the paramedics arrived. These experiences were important on two counts: I feel confident that I respond well when under pressure, and secondly the sense of satisfaction and fulfilment which came with applying knowledge and training.

<u>Paragraph 5</u>

*[Wrapping up: summary and reinforcing dedication to the subject]*
Based on my work experience in hospitals and volunteering, further academic research from books and articles in the Junior BMJ and

New Scientist, and what I learnt attending MedSim at Nottingham University and the Debate Chamber Advanced Medicine course, I am dedicated to this subject and profession. I look forward to the challenges and rewards ahead.

## EXAMPLE 2 - MEDICINE

*(NOTE: This statement is a good example of how further reading and work experience can be woven together, making the links between paragraph 2 and 3 fluid.)*

Paragraph 1

*[Reason for applying: academic engagement, fits well with outside interests]*
I want a future at university and beyond that fits best with my current interests and abilities, yet will allow me to be constantly challenged and stretched. The combination of professional skills, ethics, and deep, intellectual engagement with diverse branches of science has made Medicine my choice.

Paragraphs 2 & 3

*[Subject-specific activity 1: detailing how this increased conviction and influenced choice of course]*
Attending the Salters' Chemistry Camp and the UNIQ summer school both sharpened my academic science and laboratory skills in

a university environment, and increased my conviction that this is the right path for me. To meet the challenges in a clinical environment, I know that I first want a solid academic understanding of the human body, its processes, and treatment pathways, which I feel your degree and the way it is structured will help me achieve.

*[Subject-specific activity 2: volunteering linked to opinion and reading articles]*
When cost-cutting came into place at the care home for the elderly at which I volunteer, I saw first-hand the consequences of policy and funding shifts within the NHS, in terms of the extent and frequency of support that can be given. Visits from the physiotherapist are less frequent and a weekly memory clinic with a trained psychologist has been closed down, both of which impact on the remaining quality of life for the elderly people at the home and increase the home's reliance on volunteers like me. The medical consequences of a rapidly ageing population in the UK was further brought home in the extended feature "Billion Shades of Grey" in the Economist.

While empathy is key to patient care, I strongly believe that top-level science and a pragmatic understanding of health choice realities provide the foundation for a broader strategy, which, in turn, will improve patient care. For example, increasing the use of laparoscopic surgery, which requires focused training and research programmes, will ultimately improve patient outcomes, reduce length of hospital stay, and save money.

*[Further reading 1 and subject-specific activity 3: book trigger for arranging work experience]*
I keep up to date with big medical issues, such as euthanasia, by reading articles in the broadsheet press, e.g. The Nicklinson Case. Wanting to get a patient's view of a terminal disease and the emotional as well as physical processes they go through, I read John Diamond's "Because Cowards Get Cancer Too". This has led me to arrange a two-week placement at a local hospice (which I will complete this November) and enter a half marathon to raise money for the Marie Curie Trust.

*[Subject-specific activity 4: how work experience increased motivation to study Medicine]*
Several shifts with an Emergency Nurse Practitioner at Swansea Hospital Emergency Department underlined the strenuous hard work of medical staff. At the same time, however, I saw how the intellectual stimulation and patient interaction compensate.

*[Subject-specific activity 5: international work experience, open to new methods, culturally sensitive]*
For this coming summer, I have individually organised a summer placement at a hospital in Azerbaijan. Apart from the personal challenge of being in a country where little English is spoken, I want to experience different cultural attitudes to healthcare. I have been self-teaching myself Russian for two years, which will help at a basic level. Despite this, I will need to be flexible in my communication style and open to a very different clinical approach; both being skills which are required of the medical profession around the world and which will stand me in good stead in my future career.

Paragraph 4

*[Non subject-specific 1: showing relevant skills for course and profession]*
My interest in science is wide ranging - including being the founder of the school "Sky At Night" Society. I have been involved with the scouting movement for ten years. The responsibilities I have taken on have involved motivating, leading, and supporting others. Experiences such as taking groups of cubs from urban areas on summer country camps - both exciting and, at times, unnerving - have developed my decision-making, public-speaking, and lateral-thinking skills, all of which will be useful on this course.

Paragraph 5

*[Wrapping up: summary and confirming dedication]*
I hope that my academic ability in science, as demonstrated by my grades, my deep interest in the subject, and my proven aptitude and experience of taking care and leading others will allow me to succeed at Medicine at degree level and beyond.

## EXAMPLE 3 - MEDICINE

Paragraph 1

*[Reason for applying: trigger, plus broader academic interest in and aptitude for subject]*

It has been the more detailed study of Chemistry at A-level and beyond which has helped my decision to study Medicine at university. Learning about the processes and mechanisms of organic chemistry has underlined how it should be possible to treat the vast majority of illnesses and diseases.

Paragraph 2

*[Further reading 1: how this influenced choice of EPQ title]*
My interest has been reinforced by reading books such as "Why Chemical Reactions Happen" and "Power, Sex, Suicide", making me want to both learn more and apply my knowledge in a clinical setting. Studying Biology in parallel has given me a broader perspective, part of which involved doing the obligatory AS Biology extended coursework and an EPQ. The latter was most interesting for me because I could choose the exact parameters of the essay, "An investigation into the potential health consequences of the Paleo Diet". Self-directing my EPQ research, I referenced six scientific papers, two longitudinal studies, and numerous books and articles. I even independently arranged international phone interviews. My conclusion was that this diet has been maligned far more than the specific health results merit. I look forward to doing similar, but more demanding, research-led work at university.

*[Further reading 2: particular area of interest based on EPQ and own opinion on public health]*
The EPQ sparked my interest in the correlation between legislating against tobacco and, in the future, against sugar. I follow this debate closely in the scientific and broadsheet press. As in the 1960s,

medical opinion on the obesity epidemic in Britain is becoming increasingly politicised. As Boswell writes in "The Shape We're In", working on the frontline, doctors across many disciplines - e.g. psychology, cardiology, bariatric surgery - are urging government to see obesity as more than a matter of individual responsibility and bring out legislation that helps people stop consuming such large quantities of sugar.

Paragraph 3

*[Subject-specific activity 1: how work experience changed attitude]*
Observing a Consultant in the ENT Department at a major teaching hospital made me realise the serious implications of a procedure often considered a joke. There were several patients who wanted to have rhinoplasty. Having spoken to patients and the Consultant, I see that rhinoplasty can definitely be a necessary medical procedure for both physical and mental reasons. What seemed absurd, having to decide if the patient is really suffering or just wants cosmetic surgery at NHS expense, is now something I see as a serious budgetary and ethical decision.

*[Subject-specific activity 2: work experience opening up ethical debate]*
A two-week placement in a local Neonatal Unit introduced me to the incredibly skilled application of medicine on such tiny bodies, while highlighting the serious ethical debate which comes with the costly staff-to-patient ratio and the complex machinery required.

*[Subject-specific activity 3: competitions and how they show suitability for course]*
I have competed in several science competitions, including the team-based "Top of the Bench", the Royal Society of Chemistry Bill Bryson Prize, and the Biology Olympiad (achieving a gold medal both years). Taking part in these competitions allows me to think more creatively and apply my knowledge independently, without being helped or directed by a teacher - a beneficial experience for university study.

<u>Paragraph 4</u>

*[Non subject-specific 1: how drama has developed skills required in degree/career]*
My main interest away from academics is acting. I have taken multiple LAMDA qualifications over the past five years. Acting lead roles and public speaking in debates has given me confidence in my communication skills, and much more. Preparing for roles has taught me to how to relate to other people, trying to understand what motivates them, why they behave as they do, and how they will react to me. This has given me a strong sense of empathy, which I think will transfer well to the clinical side of Medicine. Though I am fully aware of the academic demands of Medicine as a degree and this will always come first, my goal is to continue acting at university when possible.

Paragraph 5

*[Wrapping up: reference to nature of course, and reiteration of academic interest and motivation]*
I am highly motivated by the problem-based-learning structure your Medical School provides, and hope that, with my deep-rooted academic interest, strong personal skills, and independent motivation, you see my profile as suitable for this course.

## EXAMPLE 4 - MEDICINE

Paragraph 1

*[Reason for applying: long-term career goal and academic ability]*
From the beginning of GCSEs, the sciences have been my primary academic interest and the area in which I have most excelled. As I have learned more, I have felt constrained by the school syllabus, which teaches specific "facts", only to reveal their shortcomings a year later - atom shell arrangement is a good example. To overcome this, I have pursued independent reading and research on areas I find particularly interesting (pandemics, disease vectors, childhood nutrition), while ensuring I achieve top grades in school. Looking into potential careers in virology and pandemic disease prevention and containment (including involvement in government policy) confirmed that the best first step is an undergraduate medical degree.

Paragraph 2

*[Further reading 1: independent study beyond A-level syllabus to develop own opinion]*
This interest has led me from basic texts such as Crawford's "Viruses: A Very Short Introduction" to her more complex "The Invisible Enemy" and Oldstone's "Viruses, Plagues and History". From what I have read, I believe that in our age of easy and rapid travel, the opening of economic frontier regions, such as Africa, poses significant health risks that need planning for at a global level. Whether high-profile names such as AIDS, SARS, Ebola, and Influenza, to the lesser-known MERS-CoV, it is widely accepted by the medical and political community that it is fast-mutating virus - perhaps one that makes the leap from animal to human infection - which could decimate the global population. Indeed, the statement from WHO in February 2013 that MERS-CoV was "a threat to the whole world" suggests this is probable rather than just possible.

*[Further reading 2: linking it to knowledge from other books]*
Reading articles in the New Scientist and Lancet and Wolfe's "The Viral Storm", I have closely followed the investigation trail - from Egyptian tomb bats to camels - and the higher rate person-to-person mutation.

Paragraph 3

*[Subject-specific activity 1: work experience linked to two specific areas of interest]*
Two work-experience placements, on a children's ward and at a local GP surgery, were insights into how improving children's nutrition requires engaging the whole family over a longer period of time. Doctors dealing with these issues have to be sensitive but clear on the necessary lifestyle changes for better health. These same communication skills, plus cross-cultural awareness, are needed in virus prevention, especially when working in developing countries where certain practices (burial, sexual attitudes) increase the probability of a virus spreading.

*[Subject-specific activity 2: EPQ showing independent research]*
Wanting a historic perspective on pandemics, I wrote my EPQ on "Causes of global variations in death rate in the Spanish Flu Pandemic of 1916 - 1918". For my research I used the resources of the Virology Department of Stanford University and BMJ articles. The variation of immune system response and relative strength of the 'Cytokine storm' was unexpected and reinforced how medical practitioners can take nothing for granted.

*[Subject-specific activity 3: MedSoc and interest in public health policy]*
The criticisms raised on the UK government's response to BSE, in communication and strategic planning, underline how important it is for specialised medical practitioners to help shape policy. I gave a presentation at my school's Medical Society, which I helped to

found with teacher support, on what went wrong during the BSE crisis and suggested alternative measures.

*[Subject-specific activity 4: attending open days and researching universities, showing commitment to finding right course fit]*
It is important to me to find the right academic fit for my undergraduate degree. This has involved attending multiple university medical open days, researching the type of course which will suit me (non-PBL), and selecting universities with strong Virology Departments, in the hope that I use my vacations for either volunteer or paid work experience in the labs or on research initiatives.

Paragraphs 4 & 5

*[Non subject-specific 1: long-term dedication and focus, detailing relevance for course]*
My serious hobby outside of school is karate. In five years, I have reached Brown Belt, and will be taking the Black Belt this summer. It gives me a feeling of concentration and control, which I think will help me in stressful situations in my future career. I have taken part in several regional competitions (coming first twice and third three times for my weight category) and look forward to continuing this at university as a counterpoint to my studies.

## EXAMPLE 5 - DENTISTRY

Paragraph 1

*[Reason for applying: trigger and course combines skills and interests]*
Multiple work experience placements have confirmed for me that Dentistry is the career path I wish to pursue. It combines the academic subjects I love, the precision and dexterity I am constantly developing in my activities outside of school, and interpersonal skills.

Paragraphs 2 & 3

*[Subject-specific activity 1: work experience and tenacity in getting it]*
To ensure I make the strongest application possible, my approach to preparing for it has been methodical. This has involved organising a range of work experience placements, through school contacts, family friends, and cold-calling. Three days in the Radiography Department of my local hospital was the result of six emails, two phone calls, and an informal interview. The time there was hugely informative about how to read and interpret X-rays.

*[Subject-specific activity 2: further work experience placements proving understanding of commitment involved]*
Through this contact I was introduced to a maxillofacial surgeon and will have a week of shadowing and observation next summer. My own dentist gave me his time to explain various procedures in

detail - e.g. root canal work and attaching a crown. The checking and re-checking of spacing and bite was even more important than I anticipated. Cold-calling got me an interview with a paediatric dentist specialist in Birmingham and an orthodontist. While I only had an hour with each, I prepared questions for them on the skills and challenges required in their specialism. Finally, I arranged a week's work experience last Easter at a dental laboratory, which improved my understanding of dentistry beyond the dental chair.

*[Further reading 1: wanting to understand more about details of degree]*
Prior to these experiences, I read "Dental Anatomy: Reference Guide" to get an understanding of the technical terminology and a map of the mouth, including jaw, soft tissue, and tongue, as well as teeth above and below the gums.

*[Subject-specific 3: seeking understanding of broader role of dentists]*
Wanting to understand more about dentistry and public health, I volunteered for two months with a local dental practice, accompanying a dental nurse on trips to primary schools and nurseries. The purpose of these visits (once a week, coinciding with a free morning in school) is to explain to children the importance of good dental hygiene. Having observed the dental nurse twice, I became the main presenter; an excellent way to learn how approachable you need to be when treating children.

*[Subject-specific 4: competitions showing academic ability and teamwork skills]*

Gold and silver medals at Chemistry and Biology Olympiads demonstrate my ability in science. Leading our school team to second place regionally in the National Code-breaking Challenge was satisfying on two fronts. I was able to both employ my mathematical talents in a more creative way, and to develop my skills of leadership - motivating others in the team when they found the challenge hard. I chose Business as a fourth A-level because I wanted to begin to understand the basic principles I will need in the future for my own practice or in a partnership.

Paragraph 4

*[Non subject-specific 1: tennis and its relevance for course]*
I captain my school tennis team. Though not fine motor skill, I believe this shows good hand-eye coordination and a basic ability to deal with pressure.

*[Non subject-specific 2: own business, peer mentoring, and relevant communication skills developed]*
Running my own part-time business repairing screens on iPhones and iPads for the last two years has required delicate practical skills, as well as learning how to deal with people. On work experience placements, I observed that dentists must adapt their manner to suit the patient, especially when treating children or the elderly. With customers in my own business - often older people worried about expense - I think I have developed the foundations for the clear and reassuring communication style essential to this profession. Peer mentoring in the sciences and mathematics at the school drop-in clinic, to which I give one lunchtime a week, has

helped me learn how best to motivate younger people and explain complicated ideas to them.

Paragraph 5

*[Wrapping up: commitment to course, reiterating methodical and dedicated preparation approach]*
I am confident that I have the academic ability and drive required to successfully pursue a dentistry career and hope that my commitment and focus in preparing this application over an extended period of time prove I deserve a place on your course.

## EXAMPLE 6 - VETERINARY SCIENCE

Paragraph 1

*[Reason for applying: interest and suitability, based on work experience]*
For the last four years I have been exploring in ever more depth the viability and reality of studying Veterinary Medicine and making my very strong interest into my career. After multiple work experiences: small animal practice; equine; large animals (farm); exotics; and avian, I believe I am best suited to a country practice which focuses on cattle, pigs, sheep, and poultry. The commitment required for this life's work, to the prevention of disease, animal care, and surgery in a commercial environment, is why I have spoken to as many people as possible to confirm my choice.

Paragraph 2

*[Further reading 1: linked to work experience]*
Reading Agar's "Small Animal Nutrition" tied in well with a case of feline pancreatitis I saw at my local practice where I have worked part-time for the last two years. I saw how dietary changes (low fat, high fibre) were effective in preventing relapses.

*[Further reading 2: linked to broader scientific interest / understanding]*
"Zoobiquity" by Horowitz and Bowers has helped me understand my current affairs reading on the MERS virus with its likely origins in cave bats, infecting camels, and then jumping to humans. All three being mammals is significant in the successful transfer of the virus. This is even more likely in more physiologically similar animals (e.g. dogs and wolves, humans and chimpanzees), per Wolfe's taxonomic transmission rule "the more closely related any two species are, the higher the probability that a microbe can successfully jump between them" in "The Viral Storm".

Paragraph 3

*[Subject-specific activity 1: aspect of work experience opened mind to new approaches, linking in further reading and commitment to this specific course]*
Treating equine sarcoids with the human BCG vaccine reinforced the complexity of inter-species infection and cure. Working alongside standard treatments with a specialist equine vet at a racehorse yard in Sussex, I was intrigued when told that the trainer

would bring in a holistic Reiki healer to speed up the recovery process of a foreleg fracture. The vet admitted his own past scepticism but confirmed he had seen multiple successes. This echoed what I had read about the power of placebos even on dogs in Goldacre's "Bad Science". Though I am open to new approaches to healing, I am ultimately driven by science and see animals, like humans, as bio-mechanic machines controlled by chemical processes.

*[Subject-specific activity 2: details of what further placement showed about nature of profession]*
This degree will give me a deep understanding of the processes and the tools to start a career. The farmers I met while shadowing a large animal vet for three weeks last summer contrasted significantly with my ongoing small practice work. Farmers are far more pragmatic and cost-conscious than small pet owners, whose emotional connection and unwillingness to have animals put down can be to the detriment of their animals: e.g. a vet putting drainage catheters into a dog's abdomen after liver failure and clearly limited lifespan as the owner wanted "a few more days".

*[Subject-specific activity 3: how running school society and charity work have developed relevant skills]*
Learning the emotional and communication skills to deal with wide range of human scenarios a vet faces will be stimulating. Founding and running the school Dissection Society and organising sponsorship for my charity runs have provided me with some experience of this. I have learnt to prepare younger students for the shock of actually cutting open a rat or frog, something they think

they can handle but often cannot. I have created a process whereby I speak to them individually prior to the dissection, clearly explain what is happening at each stage, and make it easy for them to leave without embarrassment if needed.

Paragraph 4

*[Non subject-specific 1: two examples of commitment to a relevant cause]*
As a hobby I enjoy running and have completed multiple 5k and 10k races and two half marathons. Though I run predominantly for fun and exercise, to date I have raised over £4,000 for the RSPCA and WWF. I volunteer weekly at the local RSPCA where I have learnt how easily animal behaviour patterns can be modified by mistreatment or caring treatment.

Paragraph 5

*[Wrapping up: summary of relevant experience, commitment to course, and motivation to make most of opportunities as an undergraduate]*
Attending university taster days and Vetsim have assured me that I can rise to the academic demands of the course, and my work experiences have proved that I will cope with the physical, mental, and emotional aspects involved. I have already looked at the opportunities available via student BVA membership and will take full advantage if offered a place.

## EXAMPLE 7 - NURSING

Paragraph 1

*[Reason for applying: well-researched choice which suits skills and interests]*

This degree in Nursing is a conscious and well-researched career decision. Having analysed what I am good at and what I enjoy over the last year, I believe that training to become a paediatric nurse unites these aspects. Completing a highly-regarded Nursing degree is the first step to achieving my goal.

Paragraphs 2 & 3

*[Subject-specific activity 1: work experience placements as a way of confirming interest in and suitability for specific area of Nursing]*

I knew at the beginning of Sixth Form that I wanted to enter a caring profession, but was unsure whether to focus on caring for children or adults. To help me identify the area which suited me best, I organised a number of work experience placements. Since then, twelve months' volunteering in both an old people's home and an under-5s play group have provided an invaluable insight into the patience and communication skills required when dealing with both groups, but it was with the children that I felt most comfortable. With them, I was able to draw on my experience of regularly helping my mother look after my two much younger brothers and of babysitting for neighbours and family friends. I feel confident I know how to entertain, relax, and control young children, even in extreme situations.

*[Further reading: own opinion formed by book and work experience]*
Reading "Call the Midwife" inspired me to set up a placement with a local district nurse. I saw that visiting people's homes is still essential for understanding in-depth how best to care for the patients, just as it was 60 years ago when Jennifer Worth glanced around her patient's room to see "bottle-feeding would be the worst thing for the baby."

*[Subject-specific activity 2: course is well-researched and current subjects at Sixth Form show suitability]*
Studying Health and Social Care, along with Psychology A-level at college has given me a good understanding of the basic topics in this course. The divide between 50% theory and 50% practical in a range of nursing environments appeals to my hands-on approach, as evidenced by my activities as part of St John's Ambulance (where I have been a member for two years). I am currently learning British Sign Language, a course I enrolled on as I think it will help with job opportunities in the future.

*[Subject-specific activity 3: further course research and proactively reaching out to relevant professionals]*
To understand more about the inter-professional nature of this degree, as outlined on the university's website, I have independently arranged meetings with two midwives and a paediatric nurse in my local area. Both reiterated that excellent communication skills are

essential within nursing, to deal with the children and their families, as well as other members of the healthcare team.

Paragraph 4

*[Non subject-specific 1: developing relevant skills through drama / public speaking]*
Knowing that they would be important for my future career, I have made a conscious effort to improve my confidence in speaking up in a group. A year ago I joined a local drama group and have had small parts in three shows performing in front of up to one hundred people. I have pushed myself to speak out more in class and this has been noted by teachers. I volunteered to give a talk to potential students and parents at the college. This went very well, which I think was due to the amount of preparation and rehearsal I put in.

*[Non subject-specific 2: relevant skills developed for course]*
Doing my Silver Duke of Edinburgh's Award has helped with leadership and decision-making skills which I have read are vital on this course. During a disagreement about map reading on our 25km hike in the Peak District, I managed to keep calm and explain why I thought a particular route was right based on two pieces of evidence (a distant farm and a high peak). This ensured the group went the right way and finished ahead of most other groups.

*[Non subject-specific 2: evidence of ability to communicate and motivate others]*
Volunteering as a Peer Mentor at a school near my college involves spending two lunchtimes a week to help Year 7 and 8 students with

mathematics. This, and my responsibilities as a Youth Leader at my local community centre, which include planning and running activities for twenty 10 to 14 year olds (music making, table tennis, video nights), have helped me relate to older children and young adolescents.

Paragraph 5

*[Wrapping up: reiterating suitability for course and motivation]*
I am a caring and compassionate person, who can get things done. I am confident about working with children and am highly motivated to do well on your course to take advantage of the opportunities it will give me, whether within the NHS or in the developing world later in my career.

Chapter 11

# CUTTING THE WORD COUNT

You are literally a few hours away from finishing your Personal Statement. Most of the hard work is behind you: doing the research; deciding on the ideas you want to put across; finding the examples you need to illustrate these ideas; setting the order in which you want to present these; and formulating the words and tone of your statement. All that is left to do is make sure there are no mistakes.

There may be light at the end of the tunnel, but this is not the time for slacking - the final stage is just as crucial as the rest. Waffling on in the first paragraph with descriptions of course content will lose the attention of admissions tutors. Spilling over the character count because you have listed too many non subject-specific hobbies will lead you to cut valuable and relevant content on books you have read. Letting just one spelling mistake slip into your statement means moving down the list of applicants.

Put simply: this is make or break time for getting an offer from your chosen university. So give yourself time to get it right. Follow each step in this chapter very carefully, and then repeat the process at least once, if not twice.

First, check that your Personal Statement is between 3,900 and 4,000 characters. Most students constantly check the character count as they go along - at first, because they think they will never have enough to say, and then because they have so much to say and do not know what to leave out. If you are still over the character limit at this stage, you need to use the following methods to make your Personal Statement more concise.

The main stylistic errors which unnecessarily lengthen your statement are:

(a) Repetition
(b) Too much description
(c) Irrelevant information
(d) Long-winded sentences

Once these errors are weeded out, your Personal Statement is likely to be down to the correct number of characters and to make a much more compelling read for admissions tutors. The examples below show you how to tackle each issue individually.

****PLAGIARISM ALERT****

*Example (Paragraph 1) -- not so good:*

"For the last four years I have been exploring in ever more depth the viability and reality of studying Veterinary Medicine and making my very strong interest into my career, just as my father and grandfather before me. From the things I have learned over these four years on multiple work experiences - small animal practice; equine; large animals (farm); exotics; and avian - I believe I am best suited to and will most enjoy and thrive in a country practice which focuses on cattle, pigs, sheep, and poultry. The commitment required for this life's work, one which my research proves I have not taken lightly, to the prevention of disease, animal care, and surgery in a commercial environment, is why I have spoken to as many people as possible to confirm my choice and career hopes."

(a) Repetition

"For the last four years I have been exploring in ever more depth the viability and reality of studying Veterinary Medicine and making my very strong interest into my career, just as my father and grandfather before me. From the things I have learned over these four years on multiple work experiences - small animal practice; equine; large animals (farm); exotics; and avian - I believe I am best suited to and will most enjoy and thrive in a country practice which focuses on cattle, pigs, sheep, and poultry. The commitment required for this life's work, one which my research proves I have not taken lightly, to the prevention of disease, animal care, and surgery in a commercial environment, is why I have spoken to as many people as possible to confirm my choice and career hopes."

*Problem 1:*
*The time taken to research and make this decision (four years) is mentioned twice.*

*Problem 2:*
*The expectation that this degree will become a career need only be stated once, at the beginning.*

(b) Too much description

"For the last four years I have been exploring in ever more depth the viability and reality of studying Veterinary Medicine and making my very strong interest into my career, just as my father and grandfather before me. From the things I have learned over these four years on multiple work experiences - small animal practice; equine; large animals (farm); exotics; and avian - I believe I am best suited to and will most enjoy and thrive in a country practice which focuses on cattle, pigs, sheep, and poultry. The commitment required for this life's work, one which my research proves I have not taken lightly, to the prevention of disease, animal care, and surgery in a commercial environment, is why I have spoken to as many people as possible to confirm my choice and career hopes."

*Problem 1:*
*It is clear that learning from these experiences enabled you to decide that this was the career for you, it does not need spelling out in such detail.*

*Problem 2:*
*The fact that you have completed so much research before making a commitment to this course proves in itself that this is a decision you have taken seriously.*

(c) Irrelevant information
"For the last four years I have been exploring in ever more depth the viability and reality of studying Veterinary Medicine and making my

very strong interest into my career, just as my father and grandfather before me. From the things I have learned over these four years on multiple work experiences - small animal practice; equine; large animals (farm); exotics; and avian - I believe I am best suited to and will most enjoy and thrive in a country practice which focuses on cattle, pigs, sheep, and poultry. The commitment required for this life's work, one which my research proves I have not taken lightly, to the prevention of disease, animal care, and surgery in a commercial environment, is why I have spoken to as many people as possible to confirm my choice and career hopes."

*Problem:*
*That members of your family have worked in this field is not relevant for admissions tutors. If anything, it detracts from your individual motivation and suggests you are just doing it because everyone else in your family has. Leave it out.*

(d) Long-winded sentences

"For the last four years I have been exploring in ever more depth the viability and reality of studying Veterinary Medicine and making my very strong interest into my career, just as my father and grandfather before me. From the things I have learned over these four years on multiple work experiences - small animal practice; equine; large animals (farm); exotics; and avian - I believe I am best suited to and will most enjoy and thrive in a country practice which focuses on cattle, pigs, sheep, and poultry. The commitment required for this life's work, one which my research proves I have not taken lightly, to the prevention of disease, animal care, and surgery in a commercial environment, is why I have spoken to as many people as possible to confirm my choice and career hopes."

*Problem:*
*All of this paragraph lacks punch. The long sentences need to be broken up and interspersed with shorter ones. The repetition should be removed and the thoughts made more concise.*

*Example (Paragraph 1) -- better:*

"For the last four years I have been exploring in ever more depth the viability and reality of studying Veterinary Medicine and making my very strong interest into my career. After multiple work experiences: small animal practice; equine; large animals (farm); exotics; and avian, I believe I am best suited to a country practice which focuses on cattle, pigs, sheep, and poultry. The commitment required for this life's work, to the prevention of disease, animal care, and surgery in a commercial environment, is why I have spoken to as many people as possible to confirm my choice."

## Chapter 12

## SPOTTING AND FIXING ERRORS

You will have read your Personal Statement hundreds of times. This can make you blind to the most straightforward mistakes. Getting someone else (if not two people) to read your Personal Statement at this final stage is absolutely essential. They will be able to spot what you no longer can. Make sure to tell them that you do not want feedback on content but instead on spelling mistakes, grammatical errors, and overall use of language.

Errors to look out for:

(a) Repetitive language
(b) Spelling mistakes / homophones (words that sound the same but mean something different when spelt differently - see examples below)
(c) Punctuation errors
(d) Lack of capitals
(e) American spelling

The examples below show you how to spot each of these errors. Follow these and then apply the same process to your own statement.

****PLAGIARISM ALERT****

*Example (Paragraph 2) -- not so good:*

"Reading Agar's "Small animal nutrition" tied in well with a case of feline pancreatitis I saw at my local practice where I have worked part-time for the last two years. I saw how dietary changes (low fat, high fibre were affective in preventing relapses. Zoobiquity by Horowitz and Bowers tied in with my analyzing of current affairs articles on the MERS virus with its likely origins in cave bats, infecting camels, and then jumping to humans. All three being mammals is significant in the successful transfer of the virus. This is even more likely in more physiologically similar animals (eg dogs and wolves, humans and chimpanzees), per Wolfe's taxonomic transmission rule "the more closely related any two species are, the higher the probability that a microbe can successfully jump between them" in "The Viral Storm"."

(a) Repetitive language

"Reading Agar's "Small animal nutrition" tied in well with a case of feline pancreatitis I saw at my local practice where I have worked part-time for the last two years. I saw how dietary changes (low fat, high fibre were affective in preventing relapses. Zoobiquity by Horowitz and bowers tied in with my analyzing of current affairs articles on the MERS virus with its likely origins in cave bats, infecting camels, and then jumping to humans. All three being mammals is significant in the successful transfer of the virus. This is even more likely in more physiologically similar animals (eg dogs and wolves, humans and chimpanzees), per Wolfe's taxonomic transmission rule “the more closely related any two species are, the higher the probability that a microbe can successfully jump between them” in “The Viral Storm”.”

*Problem:*
*The expression “tied in” is overused. There are plenty of ways round this. Take a look at the suggestions in Chapter 9 for different methods of expression. In this example, you could cut the second instance of “tied in” as it confuses rather than enhances the meaning of the sentence.*

(b) Spelling mistakes / homophones

“Reading Agar's “Small animal nutrition” tied in well with a case of feline pancreatitis I saw at my local practice where I have worked part-time for the last two years. I saw how dietary changes (low fat, high fibre were affective in preventing relapses.”

*Problem:*
*The dietary changes were “effective” not “affective”. They did not change a feeling or emotion; they had a positive impact on the health of cats.*

Classics to look out for are:

i) your / you're
ii) their / there / they're
iii) principal / principle

iv) complement / compliment
v) effect / affect
vi) who's / whose
vii) sighted / cited
viii) reining in / reigning in
ix) practice / practise
x) license / licence
xi) two / too / to
xii) altar / alter
xiii) ascent / assent
xiv) aural / oral
xv) cession / session
xvi) elicit / illicit
xvii) stationary / stationery

(c) Punctuation errors

"Reading Agar's "Small Animal Nutrition" tied in well with a case of feline pancreatitis I saw at my local practice where I have worked part-time for the last two years. I saw how dietary changes (low fat, high fibre were affective in preventing relapses. Zoobiquity by Horowitz and Bowers tied in with my analyzing of current affairs articles on the MERS virus with its likely origins in cave bats, infecting camels, and then jumping to humans. All three being mammals is significant in the successful transfer of the virus. This is even more likely in more physiologically similar animals (eg dogs and wolves, humans and chimpanzees), per Wolfe's taxonomic transmission rule "the more closely related any two species are, the higher the probability that a microbe can successfully jump between them" in "The Viral Storm"."

*Problem 1:*
*There is a bracket missing after "fibre", closing the bracket opened when referencing the dietary changes.*

*Problem 2:*
*"Zoobiquity" is the title of a book. This should be in "quotation marks".*

*Problem 3:*
*"e.g." is an abbreviation and requires full stops after each letter.*

Knowing and spotting this stuff yourself is tricky - so get someone with impeccable grammar to do it for you.

<u>(d) Lack of capitals</u>

"Reading Agar's "Small animal nutrition" tied in well with a case of feline pancreatitis I saw at my local practice where I have worked part-time for the last two years.

*Problem:*
*You are referring to the title of a book. Follow the format of the book's title, which in this case is capital letters at the beginning of each word.*

Others classics to look out for are:

i) Prefect
ii) Sixth Form
iii) Mathematics / Economics / Finance / Accounting / Politics (when you are referring to the subject to which you are applying / studying at A-level)
iv) Department (use lower case when talking about a university department in general, but upper case when referring to a specific department) - e.g. "your department's website", but "the breadth of the Management Department's contacts with international businesses"
v) Physics Society / Economics Society (a specific organisation to which you belong)
vi) University (use lower case when talking about going to "university" generally, but upper case when referring to a specific university or mentioning the details of an open day you have attended - e.g. "at the Economics Open Day at the University of Exeter".)
vii) City of London (this is a place name and therefore a proper noun with capitals at the beginnings of the words.)

(e) American spelling (highlighted in orange)

"Zoobiquity by Horowitz and Bowers tied in with my analyzing of current affairs articles on the MERS virus with its likely origins in cave bats, infecting camels, and then jumping to humans."

*Problem:*
*You are applying to a British university, so use British English. If you are not sure what is what - <u>check</u>. It should be "analysing", but better still would be to rephrase this more elegantly - see the example below.*

The classics:

i) program should be programme
ii) rigor should be rigour
iii) analyze should be analyse
iv) color should be colour
v) synthesize should be synthesise
vi) honors should be honours

*Example (Paragraph 2) -- better:*

"Reading Agar's "Small Animal Nutrition" tied in well with a case of feline pancreatitis I saw at my local practice where I have worked part-time for the last two years. I saw how dietary changes (low fat, high fibre) were effective in preventing relapses. "Zoobiquity" by Horowitz and Bowers has helped me understand my current affairs reading on the MERS virus with its likely origins in cave bats, infecting camels, and then jumping to humans. All three being mammals is significant in the successful transfer of the virus. This is even more likely in more physiologically similar animals (e.g. dogs and wolves, humans and chimpanzees), per Wolfe's taxonomic transmission rule "the more closely related any two species are, the higher the probability that a microbe can successfully jump between them" in "The Viral Storm"."

## Chapter 13

# TEACHER'S REFERENCE

As part of your UCAS application a teacher at school has to write a Teacher's Reference on your character and ability, and provide evidence of your suitability for the course and for university studies more generally. Typically, the teacher responsible for writing your report will gather mini reports from your different subject teachers, form tutor, and others who know you well, and then consolidate these into a single one page reference.

Unfortunately, not all schools ask students if there is anything they want included, nor do they let them see what has been written. Note that once the Teacher's Reference has been submitted to UCAS, you can request to see it under the Data Protection Act for a small fee.

Teachers will often have to write references for a (very) large number of students. More experienced teachers are likely to know quite a lot about certain courses for which the school's students often apply. They cannot be expected to know or have the time to research, however, the particular features of every course at every university for which their students might apply. Teachers are under great time pressure to get these references written. By proactively finding out which teacher will be writing your reference and by briefing them on the things you think relevant to your application and the course for which you are applying, you will be helping the teacher and making sure the reference you receive is as relevant and strong as possible. In other words, you can help them help you.

Two important pieces of advice:

**1. Prepare a briefing sheet**

At many of the schools I work, teachers find it extremely useful if students provide them with a <u>brief</u> summary sheet. This should include (1) the qualities the university is looking for regarding your specific course and (2) a list of your extracurricular activities (subject-specific or not) and your achievements outside of school. (Teachers may know you, but not well enough to know the details of these.) Concise bullet points work well.

**2. Timing**

Most universities give out offers on a rolling basis - first come, first served. Many students submit their applications in the second half of the application window. To secure your offers, <u>finalise your Personal Statement and submit your UCAS application early</u>.

Teachers are under a lot of pressure during this period to help everyone who is applying. Avoid the rush by giving your teacher your almost finished draft when you start back in the September of Year 13. If your school does not start the process until Year 13 (this is rare), then get it done as quickly as possible to maximise your chances. This may seem obvious, but so many students delay and delay, which ultimately lowers their chances of getting onto their preferred courses, or even of getting any offer at all. <u>You can be smarter than them and beat the competition to get your top choice</u>.

## Chapter 14

# OTHER HURDLES TO UNIVERSITY ADMISSIONS

Your Personal Statement is finished (well done!), but you have not yet secured a university offer. There is more to come.

Every year at the schools I attend, there are students who have not spent enough time looking at the entry requirements for each of their five chosen universities. Many check only their favourite choice and assume the rest will be the same. This means that they simply do not know about required admission tests, interviews, or submitted work, and, as a result, do not get the results they could have in these because they were underprepared. Read the requirements and give yourself time to prepare.

A few pointers to help you along the way.

### 1. GCSE Requirements

Many courses have minimum GCSE grade requirements. Every year I meet students who have one or two of their applications rejected without even being properly checked or the Personal Statement read because they selected a university where they do not meet the basic GCSE requirements. If you fall into this trap, you are simply wasting an opportunity. Please check carefully.

## 2. Admissions Tests

More and more universities are using admission tests (e.g. UKCAT, BMAT, ELAT, PAT, HAT, and TSA) to filter the increasing numbers of high quality students applying. Most prospective medics, dentists, and vets will have to take either the BMAT, UKCAT, or both. The preparation strategy many students employ is not useful. For tests held in November, students often think that doing minimal preparation over the summer holidays is fine, as they will put in all the hours needed over the autumn half term. This is simply not enough. The best preparation is extensive and enduring, i.e. every day for half an hour in the summer holidays.

Many tutoring services offer focused day-long courses on preparing for this test. Completing one of these either before or during the summer holidays is definitely worthwhile.

## 3. Interviews

It is very likely if you are applying for Medicine, Dentistry, or Veterinary Medicine that you will be called to an interview. Some universities will interview for Nursing. There are many types of interview, from the formal and intense Oxbridge interviews or the multiple mini-interviews (including role playing actors) for Medicine, to the softer "we would like you to come and have a look around the faculty and have a chat" type interviews.

For one-on-one interview preparation, contact me via my website: www.gwynday.com. This training can be done in person anywhere in the world or by Skype, depending on your preference. Alternatively, I work with Oxbridge Applications at several group events around the country each autumn.

## 4. Submitted Work

This is mainly required by Oxbridge Colleges. If you do need to submit an essay, or in some cases two, there is one vital piece of advice - check the criteria. When doing so be aware of two critical points: (1) the type of essay required (e.g. coursework, a competition essay, an essay written under exam conditions), and (2) the exact type of phrasing required in the essay question (e.g. comparative, textual analysis, summary). Every year I hear from students who have realised too late that they have submitted the "wrong type" of essay and only fully read the criteria on the university website after they have been rejected. You can be smarter than that.

## Appendix 1

# FURTHER SUPPORT (www.gwynday.com)

The decisions you make during Sixth Form are crucial to your future academic and professional success. I offer a range of one-on-one advice covering Personal Statements, interviews, and future career shaping. If you feel you would benefit from any or all of these services, contact me via my website (www.gwynday.com) to discuss rates and timeframes. This is your chance to stand out.

### ONE-ON-ONE PERSONAL STATEMENT COACHING

My Personal Statement Coaching includes unlimited advice, corrections, editing, and proofreading until you are happy with your Personal Statement. As part of the service I offer a money-back guarantee. So if you do not get a university offer, I will give you your money back.

### INTERVIEW PREPARATION

I am used by some of the top schools in the UK and internationally to prepare their students for interviews. Taking up my one-on-one Interview Preparation, you can get personalised training. I use the real questions asked in previous years and my NLP expertise to develop your ability to structure, consider, analyse, and, above all, demonstrate intelligent thinking in the pressure cooker that is the interview (or interviews).

## THE SIXTH-FORM PROGRAMME

The Programme is specially designed to ensure that you are in the strongest position from Sixth Form onwards to beat the competition. In this process, I help you choose the best course and university for you; guide your further reading and extracurricular activities; tailor university and internship application material to leverage the work you have put in; work with you to prepare for admissions tests; and hone your communication skills for interview. With my guidance, you will be sure to get where you want to go, both academically and professionally, at university and beyond.

## Appendix 2

# READING LIST

The books mentioned in Chapter 5, plus a few additional reading ideas:

### Medicine

"The Oxford Handbook of Clinical Diagnosis"
"The Emperor of All Maladies: A Biography of Cancer" by Siddhartha Mukherjee
"The Man Who Mistook His Wife for a Hat" by Oliver Sacks
"How We Live" by Sherwin B. Nuland
"Mutants: On Genetic Variety and the Human Body" by Armand Marie Leroi
"The Epigenetics Revolution: How modern biology is rewriting our understanding of genetics, disease and inheritance" Nessa Carey
"Philosophy of Biology" by Michael Ruse
"Why Chemical Reactions Happen" by James Keeler and Peter Wothers
"Power, Sex, Suicide: Mitochondria and the Meaning of Life" by Nick Lane
"Because Cowards Get Cancer" by John Diamond
"The Viral Storm: The Dawn of a New Pandemic Age" by Nathan Wolfe
"The Shape We're In" by Sarah Boseley

## Dentistry

See above for Medicine
"Bad Science" by Ben Goldacre
"Dental Anatomy: Reference Guide"
"The Complete Pre-Dental Guide to Modern Dentistry" by John Syrbu
"The Excruciating History of Dentistry: Toothsome Tales & Oral Oddities from Babylon to Braces" by James Wynbrandt

## Veterinary Science

"Essential Cell Biology" by Alberts et al.
"Life at the Extremes" by Frances Ashcroft
"Biomedicine and the Human Condition: Challenges, Risks, and Rewards" by Michael G. Sargent
"Life on Earth" by David Attenborough (TV series)
"The Viral Storm: The Dawn of a New Pandemic Age" by Nathan Wolfe

## Nursing

"The Spirit Catches You and You Fall Down: A Hmong Child, Her American Doctors, and the Collision of Two Cultures" by Anne Fadiman
"Call the Midwife" by Jennifer Worth

“Notes on Nursing: What It Is and What It Is Not” by Florence Nightingale
“Critical Care: A New Nurse Faces Death, Life, and Everything in Between” by Theresa Brown
“The Student Nurse Handbook: A Survival Guide” by Bethann Siviter
“Ross and Wilson Anatomy and Physiology of Health and Illness” by Anne Waugh

17765565R00108

Printed in Great Britain
by Amazon